THE
PCOS
NUTRITION CENTER
COOKBOOK

100 Easy and Delicious
Whole Food Recipes to Beat PCOS

Written by Angela Grassi
and Natalie Zaparzynski

The PCOS Nutrition Center Cookbook:
100 Easy and Delicious Whole Food Recipes to Beat PCOS

Written by Angela Grassi and Natalie Zaparzynski

Copyright © 2014 Angela Grassi
Luca Publishing
14 S. Bryn Mawr Avenue, Suite 204, Bryn Mawr, PA 19010
(484) 252-9028
www.PCOSnutrition.com

Cover and interior design by Ciara Christine
Edited by Juliann Schaeffer
Cover photo by Marilyn Barbone

ISBN: 978-0-9851164-3-9

This cookbook is dedicated to those who
enjoy eating whole foods. May you have
a lifetime of good health.

Acknowledgements

Developing this cookbook was a lot of fun but also a lot of effort. We would like to recognize the many individuals who inspired, supported, and mentored us along the way. Thank you to dietitian and cookbook coach Maggie Green for helping to get this project going and for all your valuable advice. Thank you to Juliann Schaeffer for filling in at the final moment and for giving this cookbook the finishing touches that it needed. Thank you to Omar Aziz for his hard work coding this cookbook for the many platforms it's featured in. A special thank you to Ciara Christine for all your hard work designing such a fantastic cover for this cookbook that fits in line perfectly with our vision of whole food ingredients, and for doing an amazing job with the interior design. I couldn't have asked for better. Thank you for your flexibility and patience with us along the way.

Being dietitians, we are fortunate to have so many friends who are also dietitians and who can really cook in the kitchen! Thank you to all the fabulous women who have shared their delicious recipes with us. Susan Adams, thank you for sharing your Carrot Coriander Soup and Spicy Orange Chicken with Carrots and Broccoli recipes with us. They are so delicious! Thank you Susan Dopart for the great care you provide your patients with PCOS and diabetes, and for sharing your yummy Pork with Apples and Carrots recipe from your terrific book *A Recipe for Life from by The Doctor's Dietitian.* To my long-time friend and dietitian Moira Gledhill who has never prepared me a meal that was less than fabulous, thank you for sharing your Spicy Cilantro Lime Chicken and Marinated Flank Steak recipes. They do not disappoint!

We want to thank Stephanie Mattei from the Center for Acceptance and Change for once again agreeing to contribute your time to another PCOS book. Thank you for sharing your delicious family favorite Grilled Chicken Thighs recipe. You are an amazing superwoman! Thank you Teresa Grassi for sharing your delicious favorite recipe, Savory Turkey Breast and for all her love and support. And thank you to Maiah Miller our cookbook contest winner for sharing your yummy and creative Mini Quinoa Kale Quiches recipe with us.

Finally, thank you to all of our family and friends who we have subjected to taste testing (whether they wanted to or not!) or who have prepared some of our recipes themselves. Thank you for your honest feedback so we could make this cookbook the best that it can be.

Angela's Acknowledgments:

A special thank you to my co-author Natalie Zaparzynski for signing on to do this project with me and for all your hard work developing such delicious, healthy recipes. From the moment I met you, I saw the passion you had for food and cooking and for helping women with PCOS. I'm looking forward to more projects together.

At an early age, I was exposed to the fun and challenge of cooking from recipes while watching my mom and her best friend and neighbor Donna Grant prepare meals from Bon Appétit Magazine. Some of the recipes they made came out better than others, some looking and tasting just as good as the cover. Thank you to my mom and Donna for showing me that no matter how a recipe comes out, cooking it was the fun part. Thank you also for your constructive criticism with these recipes.

Finally, I would like to thank my family for their love and support with yet another book so soon after the last one. Thank you to my son Henry for tasting everything I put in front of you and for your patience sharing me with the writing of this cookbook. Luca, who by watching his mom write her cookbook, inspired you to write your own cookbook, I am beyond flattered that you want to be an author like me. Thank you for your enthusiasm and support of this book. Finally, I'd like to thank Chris. How lucky I am to be married to everyone's favorite guy. I can't thank you enough for your support, encouragement, and help editing, tasting and even developing an award winning recipe (Mango Pineapple Salsa!) for this cookbook. I love you.

Natalie's Acknowledgments:

A big thank you to my family and friends for taste-testing and critiquing my recipes during this year. Especially to my husband, Zach. You are the best sous chef and dish washer I could ask for. Your encouragement and support throughout my dietetic journey has meant so much. I especially thank you for eating whatever healthy dish I put in front of you, without complaint. I know it's not easy being a dietitian's husband!

Table of Contents

Introduction

Meal Plans

Shopping List

Breakfast

Soups

Salads

Sandwiches

Main

Meatless Main

Sides/Vegetables

Introduction

"Let food be your medicine and medicine be your food." Such sage advice was attributed to Hippocrates so many centuries ago, but it still applies to today's tech-savvy and processed food-heavy society. Hippocrates surely wasn't referring to the plight of polycystic ovary syndrome (PCOS) in particular when he uttered those words, but yet women with PCOS are uniquely suited to benefit from this advice because of their unique concerns stemming from how PCOS intertwines reproductive and metabolic hormones.

So often we've found that women with PCOS are overfed and undernourished. They eat sufficient calories to sustain them but not quality foods to properly fuel their bodies. As a result, they often suffer from a barrage of symptoms, from uncomfortable blood sugar crashes and sweet tooth cravings to exhausting migraines and fertility struggles. Yet these, along with constant fatigue, mood swings, and nutritional deficiencies, can all be aided (if not corrected) by simply eating the right foods.

No, there is currently no cure for PCOS, but it can be managed—and diet and lifestyle changes are actually two of the best ways to do just that (they're also the primary approaches used by clinicians to treat PCOS). Studies have shown that when women with PCOS improved the quality of their diets, they saw positive changes in glucose, insulin, cholesterol, androgens (male sex hormones), female sex hormones, blood pressure, and fertility. What does that mean exactly? In simple terms, when PCOS patients ate the right foods, they improved their health.

Not only is diet a way to remedy PCOS symptoms, it's paramount to preventing further, more destructive complications. The harsh reality is that if not managed sufficiently, PCOS can lead to chronic diseases such as heart disease, cancer, and type 2 diabetes. Most women with PCOS show an intrinsic insulin resistance, and this resistance increases the risk for both diabetes and heart disease and it also contributes to infertility. Compared with women of the same weight, women with PCOS have been shown to have higher insulin levels than women without the condition—and that applies to all women with PCOS, whether thin, overweight, or somewhere in between. Having high insulin levels is an independent risk factor for developing diabetes. An alarming study published in Diabetes showed that the prevalence of type 2 diabetes in middle-aged women with PCOS was 6.8 times higher than that of the general female population of similar age. As such, adopting a healthful diet for the long term is not only necessary to improve the health of women with PCOS but perhaps prevent the onset of these chronic conditions in the long run.

There's no question that improving your diet can prevent further medical complications, boost fertility, and optimize your health. And there's no better time than the present to start changing how you eat to reap these benefits. To get you started, we've compiled a short summary for you to better understand how different foods affect PCOS. Learning how certain foods affect insulin levels and which foods will help vs. hurt you will help you not just enjoy the recipes in this cookbook but also understand how to make better overall food choices as a woman with PCOS, wherever you are.

Carbohydrate Foods

Bread and pasta may be the first foods to come to mind when most people think "carbs," but in addition to grains, carbohydrate food sources can also come in the guise of fruits, vegetables, milk, beans, and legumes. Even more important than identifying them is noting that not all carbohydrates are created equally. As some carbs will cause glucose and insulin to spike faster than others, a carbohydrate can either promote insulin resistance (and weight gain) or fight it (and aid weight loss).

The glycemic index (GI), which has a scale from 0 (lowest) to 100 (highest), is a great tool to help you determine which carbohydrates are best for you. In general, foods with a high GI value will cause a more rapid increase in blood sugar levels, requiring more insulin to be secreted. In simple terms, this translates to more insulin resistance and a harder time keeping your weight in check. Low GI foods, on the other hand, digest more slowly in the body and tend to avoid those dramatic glucose and insulin spikes. A more balanced blood sugar means an easier time balancing PCOS symptoms. For those with PCOS, overweight or not, low GI (whenever possible) is the way to go.

While the GI index can be a useful tool (you can find more information on certain foods at glycemicindex.com), no one expects you to memorize the GI specifics for the hundreds of foods you eat each month. Instead, we advise a simple alternative: Eat predominately "slow carbs," or whole grains and other high-fiber foods that take some time to digest and thus have a lower GI value. To help you determine what those foods look like, we've broken down what some of the most common carbohydrate categories look like—and what they mean for women with PCOS.

Simple carbohydrates are carbohydrates broken down into very refined or tiny glucose particles (meaning the body doesn't have to work very hard to break them down for energy). Because of this, these foods enter the bloodstream immediately and cause a rapid rise in blood sugar, which triggers a rapid increase in insulin. Eating simple carbohydrates worsens PCOS by raising insulin levels and contributing to weight gain. Simple carbohydrates wreak havoc in a PCOS body, so do your best to eliminate simple carbohydrates from your diet, wherever possible.

Examples of simple carbohydrate foods include candy, baked goods, sweetened beverages (i.e., soda, iced tea, juice), and sugar.

Refined carbohydrates are similar to simple carbohydrates, but they require slightly more processing during digestion to be used as energy. Because refined carbohydrates don't contain fiber or the nutrient profile of a whole grain, they offer little nutritional value. Like simple carbohydrates, refined carbs raise insulin levels as they enter the blood-stream, causing a rapid surge in insulin and subsequent worsening insulin resistance. The first ingredient in these typically processed products often reads "enriched wheat flour." These carbohydrates are also no friend of women with PCOS and should be avoided whenever possible.

Examples of refined carbs include white rice, white flour, white bread, bagels, and low-fiber sweetened cereals.

Unrefined or whole-grain carbohydrates take an even longer time to digest, which means these are the best type of grains for women with PCOS to eat. Eating these types of foods can improve insulin resistance by slowing the release of glucose and thus preventing large insulin spikes. The minerals found in whole grains, such as chromium, magnesium, and selenium, may also help benefit insulin levels. These nutrients, along with dietary fiber, phytochemicals, and antioxidants—all found in whole grains—may help lower blood pressure and decrease the risk of heart disease and diabetes. And the fiber in whole grains can help with weight management, as these items are typically more filling. To balance these types of foods with others, keep the portion size of them to about a quarter of your plate.

Examples of whole grains include oats, spelt, millet, brown rice, wheat berries, and quinoa. Most pastas have a low GI, but try out whole wheat pasta made with durum semolina flour and cook al dente. This lowers the GI even more. Most breads, even whole grain ones, have a high GI, so we suggest using sprouted grain or sourdough breads, which have lower GI values.

Fruits contain carbohydrates, yes, but they also provide important vitamins, minerals, antioxidants, and fiber that offer numerous benefits, such as lowering blood pressure, insulin, and cholesterol, and even cancer prevention. To get the most benefit without too many carbs, try to choose fruits with the skin on them (such as apples, blueberries, and strawberries). These tend to have a lower GI than fruits eaten without the skin (such as pineapple and watermelon). Be sure to avoid fruit juice altogether, as this will quickly spike insulin levels.

Vegetables, as with fruit, also provide numerous health benefits, due to their high fiber content and rich supply of vitamins, minerals, and antioxidants. Vegetables' benefits mirror those offered by fruits, including improving blood pressure, cholesterol, and insulin numbers and potentially preventing cancer. While vegetables offer a wealth of wholesomeness, the type of vegetable (starchy or nonstarchy) is of particular importance to those with PCOS.

Starchy vegetables have a higher carbohydrate content and contribute to raising insulin levels more than nonstarchy ones. Examples of starchy vegetables include corn and potatoes. While these are higher in carbohydrates than nonstarchy vegetables, starchy vegetables are still nutritious and can be part of a balanced diet (just keep the serving size of them to that of a quarter of your plate).

Nonstarchy vegetables include broccoli, zucchini, spinach, green beans, and peppers. Due to these foods' low-carbohydrate content, eating nonstarchy vegetables will not cause the greater spikes in insulin that comes with eating starchy vegetables. Nonstarchy vegetables are full of fiber but low in calories, so you should feel free to eat them to your delight (and meal satisfaction).

Legumes consist of lentils, beans, and peas. Legumes are low on the GI scale, provide a good source of plant-based proteins, and are rich in fiber, folate, iron, and other important vitamins and minerals that improve insulin.

Milk is a rich source of calcium and protein and is also considered a carbohydrate due to its high lactose content. There is evidence that milk, in particular nonfat milk, can contribute to increasing androgen and insulin levels. For these reasons, we recommended women with PCOS limit their dairy intake coming from yogurt or milk to two or fewer servings per day.

Protein-Containing Foods

Protein, which provides essential fuel to the human body, is much more a friend to the PCOS body than most carbohydrates. In general, proteins by themselves don't require much insulin and don't raise insulin levels like carbohydrates do. Eating protein with meals and snacks can actually add fullness and help stabilize blood sugar levels throughout the day. Protein-containing foods that come from animal sources include meat, poultry, pork, fish, seafood, eggs, and dairy, whereas plant-based proteins include legumes, nuts, and soy.

A note about soy-based foods: Soy-based proteins include soy milk, tofu, and edamame. To date, the evidence regarding how soy consumption benefits women with PCOS has thus far been mixed. One study has shown that the use of soy in women with PCOS not only reduced LDL cholesterol but also significantly reduced luteinizing hormone, triglycerides, and testosterone. However, a larger study showed that high intake of soy can affect fertility. Until more research is done on the influence of soy on reproduction and other parameters, it may be beneficial to limit soy to a few servings each week and choose fermented types of soy (like tempeh and miso) when possible. Also, choose soy foods that are not genetically modified (non-GMO).

Fats and Oils

Once vilified for contributing to weight gain and other health problems, dietary fats are now known to be an important aspect of overall health and well-being. Because of the unique mouth feel and palatability fats provide to meals, diets containing too little fat can often contribute to overeating or bingeing since they can make you feel hungrier and less satisfied.

Dietary fat doesn't require insulin because it doesn't break down into glucose, but this doesn't mean you should eat it in unlimited quantities. Eating too much saturated fat (from beef, poultry, and full-fat dairy) and trans fats (from hydrogenated oils in processed baked and fried foods) has been shown to increase the risk for heart disease. When it comes to fats, it's not just how much you eat but what kind that really makes the most difference.

Eating the right balance of fatty acids is particularly important for the treatment, prevention, and maintenance of inflammation, which is commonly found in PCOS. Eating too many omega-6 fats, the type you should limit when possible, is associated with heart attacks, stroke, arthritis, osteoporosis, inflammation, mood disorders, and certain types of cancer. Omega-6 fatty acids are unsaturated fats found in vegetable oils such as palm, soybean, corn, safflower, cottonseed, grapeseed, and sunflower oil. These fats are also found in margarine, some meats and poultry, baked goods, breads, crackers, and salad dressings. You can spot (and then avoid) them by checking the ingredient list for palm, soybean, corn, safflower, cottonseed, or sunflower oil.

Conversely, monounsaturated fats, which are the mainstays of the Mediterranean diet, include olive oil, olives, nuts, nut butters, and seeds. Monounsaturated fats are cardio protective. These fats can help reduce bad cholesterol levels in your blood and lower your risk of heart disease and stroke. Overall, monounsaturated fats are much better for you and, as such, most of the recipes in this cookbook call for olive oil and incorporate a variety of monounsaturated fats.

And lastly, omega-3s are another type of fat that are essential to humans and offer numerous health benefits to women with PCOS. In particular, they can help improve mood, cholesterol, insulin, and inflammation, and they can even provide better hair and skin quality. In regard to fertility, omega-3 fats have been shown to improve egg quality and ovulation and are necessary for a healthy pregnancy. The main sources of omega-3s include fatty types of fish such as tuna, trout, and wild salmon. Nonfish sources include avocados, walnuts, seeds, and egg yolks. We recommend including omega-3-containing foods in your diet on a regular basis, and *The PCOS Nutrition Center Cookbook* offers many recipes that will help you accomplish that.

Now, we know that was a lot of information. And we don't expect you to remember it all in one shot. That's why we created these recipes—to help you put these recommendations into practice. The recipes and meal plans created for this book are consistent with the recommendations for the optimal diet for women with PCOS. That includes all the good things discussed above, including healthy fats, slow whole grains, and plenty of fruits and vegetables—without all the stuff that can wreak havoc on PCOS (such as refined grains and trans fats). All of these recipes are low in both saturated fat and sodium but high in the flavor that you need to live well and eat deliciously with PCOS. With your newfound know-how and this recipe guide in hand, we hope you will rediscover the pleasure and fun of making and eating food that is both good and good for you.

About This Cookbook

For this cookbook's creation, we thank the many women with PCOS who we've counseled at the PCOS Nutrition Center and come to know through the years. They continually came to us for delicious and healthy recipes to feed themselves and their families. For years, women have been asking us for a collection of PCOS-friendly (and easy!) recipes that they could prepare at home. As we can attest firsthand, integrating PCOS into one's life is an overwhelming job in itself; learning to plan and prepare the right foods for PCOS can create even more stress.

A quick Internet search for PCOS and nutrition can bring a hodgepodge of incorrect and misguided advice that's not based on scientific evidence, and this can result in even more confusion.

To help women with PCOS take back their mealtime sanity as well as their health, we've taken the guesswork out of the equation by creating recipes that are not only delicious but fine-tuned to beat PCOS. Even better, we've developed a four-week meal plan using the recipes in this cookbook and added all the ingredients together in a convenient shopping list. We've done the work to help you eat great so you can feel even better for it.

Whole foods can heal PCOS

This isn't a diet cookbook. Eating well isn't about dieting but learning to enjoy food and choosing the right options to nourish our bodies. Make no mistake: Whole foods can heal PCOS. What makes a food "whole"? Whole foods relate to any foods that are unprocessed and contain no added sugars, additives, or artificial sweeteners and substances. Think of them as foods in their natural state (an apple picked straight from the tree, a peanut picked from the ground). Examples of whole foods that you will see in our recipes include fruits, vegetables, beans, lentils, and whole grains such as quinoa, brown rice, and oats. We focus so much on whole foods because they contain the vitamins and minerals, fiber, and antioxidants that can beat PCOS.

All too often we find women with PCOS are more focused on the foods they can't eat rather than the foods they can. We hope this guide helps you uncover the plethora of foods that are available to you that will not only taste great but will improve your health. Take vegetables, for instance. Government guidelines advise us to consume 1 ½ to 2 cups of fruit and 2 ½ cups of vegetables each day to maximize our health. Most individuals don't meet these requirements, yet simply eating more fruits and vegetables alone can do wonders to improve your PCOS. This was confirmed by one study in which overweight women with PCOS who followed the Dietary Approaches to Stop Hypertension (DASH) eating plan lost abdominal fat and showed significant improvements in insulin resistance and inflammation markers. The DASH diet is designed to be rich in fruits, vegetables, whole grains, and low-fat dairy products and low in saturated fats, cholesterol, refined grains, sodium, and sweets. (The recipes in this cookbook, along with our four-week meal plans, are consistent with these guidelines.) Likewise, eating more of the healthier sources of fats like olive oil, nuts, avocados, seeds, and fish can help beat PCOS as well.

All of the recipes featured in this cookbook are PCOS-friendly and focus on a variety of whole foods, slow or low-glycemic index grains that won't spike insulin levels, healthy fats, fruits, vegetables—and flavor! So much flavor. Best of all, we've provided the nutrition facts for each recipe so you can see exactly what's in each. This is especially important if you're tracking calories, carbohydrates, fat, or sodium amounts. We're hoping knowing the nutrition facts will also help you plan your meals according to your (and your family's) unique needs.

You don't need to be an expert chef to prepare the recipes in this cookbook. If you aren't an experienced cook, please take heart: You will find that with practice and time, your confidence in the kitchen will only improve. Sometimes using fresh, high-quality ingredients means more than any skill, and they can take your meals to a whole new level. That's one of our favorite things about this cookbook—it uses fresh, whole foods and herbs instead of large amounts of salt or sugar for flavor. Leave any caution at the door and just trust us that using new ingredients, such as cooking with different grains, using tempeh, or trying out a variety of herbs, spices, or vegetables, will only add creativity and fun to the cooking process.

When we were fleshing out these recipes, our vision was to keep this cookbook as simple as possible. In truth, we know how it feels to come home from a long and stressful day and be greeted by hungry mouths with no plan (or energy) to make a meal come together. That's why we worked to keep the meal preparation time down and made the dishes easy to pull together. As you will see in the meal plans we created, any recipes that do require a little more time than others are planned for weekends. To note, if any recipe heats up more than the crowd you're serving, save any extra for another night or simply freeze (up to three months) for future meals.

The Benefits of Home-cooking

When we eat meals outside of the home, we are exposing ourselves to uncontrolled (and often unknown) amounts of sugar, salt, and fat. The best and quickest way to improve the quality of your diet is to prepare more of your meals at home. When you cook your own food, not only can you cater to your own tastes and preferences, but you also know exactly what is going into each dish, including sodium, fat, salt, and sugar amounts. Another important benefit is the priceless face time with friends and family members that comes from cooking and eating a self-prepared meal together.

Cooking is Mindful

By definition, mindfulness is a mental state achieved by focusing on the awareness of the present moment while calmly acknowledging and accepting feelings, thoughts, and bodily sensations. While some may find the idea of cooking a stressful experience or another job to do, we suggest looking at cooking as an opportunity to practice mindfulness. Consider the preparation for a stir-fry. Chopping vegetables requires your full, undivided attention—without it, you could easily cut yourself. Stir-frying vegetables requires mindfulness as well. If you don't focus on moving around the vegetables in the hot pan, they will burn. We encourage you to look at the process of cooking as a mindful experience and hope this will increase your mindfulness with (and enjoyment of) other daily activities.

Where's the Sugar?

The recipes in this cookbook contain little or no added sugar. Most nutrition analysis programs, such as the one we use for our recipes (**Foodworks**), only calculate total sugars, which include natural ones (sugar found in fruit) plus added ones (such as sugar or honey). This is consistent with a food package's Nutrition Facts Panel. The best way to check if a certain food contains sugar is to look at the ingredients list on the package. Look for words like syrup, sugar, dextrose, honey, or fructose. The lower sugar is on the ingredient list, the less amount is added to a product. To tell how much sugar is in a recipe, look at the amounts and sources of sugars being used.

The hormone insulin is an appetite stimulant, which means it increases cravings for sugary foods. This explains why so many women with PCOS report intense, almost urgent cravings for sweets, even just after finishing a meal. The best way to manage these cravings is to limit the amount of sugar in your diet. The less sugar you have, the less you will want it. This is why you won't see dessert recipes featured in this cookbook. While we don't recommend daily desserts, we do understand (and appreciate ourselves) that sweets are a pleasure to be enjoyed in moderation. As such, we include chocolate, especially dark chocolate containing 70% or higher cocoa as it contains antioxidants, in our four-week meal plans, but stress moderate amounts in this or other sweet treats.

What to Drink?

The Institute of Medicine recommends most adult women need an average of 9 cups of fluid each day. As with food, not all beverages are created equal, for taste and especially health.

We recommend getting most of your fluid from water itself, but a morning cup of coffee (or two) is OK, too. Even better, make one of those cups of tea, as studies have shown drinking tea may help improve PCOS symptoms. Spearmint tea, for example, has been shown to have anti-androgen effects in PCOS and can reduce hirsutism. And green tea has anti-inflammatory properties. You will see matcha, a type of green tea, used as an ingredient in some of the smoothie recipes in this cookbook.

We recommend avoiding all juices, sodas, and other caloric beverages because of their dramatic effect on raising insulin levels. While beverages containing artificial sweeteners don't appear to affect glucose levels, the effect on insulin levels isn't clear. For this reason, we recommend women with PCOS avoid artificially sweetened beverages. With the exception of moderate consumption of red wine which has antioxidants, we advise avoiding alcoholic beverages.

Plates for Easy Portion Control

We recommend each balanced meal contain part protein, whole grains, and vegetables. To help you determine how much of each you should be eating at one time, there's no fancy tools required—all you really need is your plate. To use the plate method for portion control, simply divide your plate in half. Fill one whole half with nonstarchy vegetables, such as leafy greens or broccoli. One-quarter of the other half should contain a lean protein source, such as fish or chicken. The last quarter should be filled with whole grains. A balanced meal is as simple as that!

Suggested Kitchen Tools

To make the recipes in this cookbook, we've compiled a list of suggested kitchen tools to make the cooking process go smoothly:

- **Good quality knives**
- **Cutting boards**
- **Measuring cups and spoons**
- **Whisk and mini whisk**
- **Mixing bowls (small, medium, large)**
- **Serving bowls (small, medium, large)**
- **Serving utensils**
- **Cast iron skillet**
- **Nonstick skillet**
- **Cooking pots (small, medium, stockpot)**
- **Food processor**
- **Microplane**
- **Garlic press**
- **Stainless steel fish grill plate**
- **Fish spatula**
- **Stainless steel or wood skewers**
- **Grill or grill pan**
- **Food thermometer**
- **Pepper grinder**
- **Citrus juicer**

Food Safety Advice

Food-borne illnesses (commonly known as food poisoning) can be very serious, even deadly. To minimize your risk of developing a food-borne illness, the United States Department of Agriculture recommends the following advice:

- Wash your hands and surfaces often.

- Avoid cross-contamination by keeping raw meat, poultry, seafood, and eggs away from ready-to-eat foods.

- Keep your refrigerator temperature at 40°F or below and freezer 0°F or below.

- Never thaw frozen food on the counter top. Instead, defrost food in the refrigerator, in cold water, or in the microwave.

▶ Use a food thermometer to ensure the food is cooked to a safe internal temperature (see chart below).

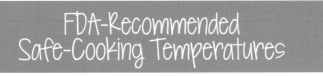

FDA-Recommended Safe-Cooking Temperatures

Ground Meat & Meat Mixtures

Beef, pork, veal, lamb	160°F
Turkey, chicken	165°F

Poultry

Chicken & turkey whole	165°F
Poultry Parts	165°F
Duck & goose	165°F

Ham

Fresh, raw	160°F
Precooked (to reheat)	140°F

Eggs

Cook until yolk & white are firm	
Egg dishes	140°F

Seafood

Fish	145°F
(or flesh is opaque & separates easily with fork)	
Seafood	opaque and firm

Leftovers & casseroles	165°F

Source: FDA

Grocery Shopping Tips

Unlike what some may think (and what many have likely experienced), food shopping doesn't have to be a dreaded task. The tips below will help you breeze through the grocery store with a smile, finding both affordable and healthful food options in a snap. For your convenience, we've provided a shopping list for you to use with our four-week meal plans.

Stick to the store's outer perimeter
This is where the majority of the best whole foods are located, protein-containing meats, fish, and cheeses as well as fresh, unprocessed foods such as fruits and vegetables. Skip the middle aisles as much as possible to avoid putting too many processed foods in your cart.

Don't shop when you're hungry
It's totally true: When we're hungry, our blood sugar lowers and everything (and we mean everything) looks great. Not only will you put more food in your cart, but you'll also end up spending more money when you shop on an empty stomach. Try to shop shortly after a meal whenever possible.

Look carefully at expiration dates
There's nothing more irritating than getting home from a tense grocery shopping trip to find that one of the foods you just bought will expire the next day. Spending a little extra time on this now could save you lots later. When selecting a food product, look for one that has the longest expiration date of all the others on the shelf. This may require a bit of hunting through items, but it'll ensure your food is freshest when you buy it and will stay freshest the longest.

Make a shopping list with a meal plan for at least three days
With long lines (and possibly little hands who want to help), grocery shopping can be a daunting task on a good day. Doing it without a plan will make it even harder. Before heading for the grocery store, ask yourself what meals you will be making in the next several days. Write them down, along with the food items that you need that week. Go through each meal, starting with breakfast, listing all the ingredients you'll need. (If desired, search through your coupons and use the store circular for extra savings.) To make this easier, our convenient weekly shopping lists include all the ingredients needed to prepare recipes for each week of the meal plan.

Examine the labels
Before putting food in your cart, carefully read food labels. For canned goods, look for the label "BPA-free." Choose foods labeled "organic" and "non-GMO." Watch out for foods high in saturated or trans fats, sodium, or sugar. For processed items, look for foods where the first ingredient reads "whole" and contains at least 3 grams or more of fiber per serving. If possible, compare the food item to others in the aisle to make the healthiest choice possible.

Buy local whenever possible
Buying food that didn't sit in transit for an extended time will often be fresher (and taste better!) and can contain less or no pesticides or fertilizers. These choices are also environmentally friendly, and if it takes you to a local farmers' market, where most local foods are sold, you'll get the bonus of meeting and connecting with other community members as well as local farmers.

Avoid the most crowded shopping times
You're likely to be more frustrated and feel more rushed to get out of the store when it's crowded. These feelings could result in spontaneous (and expensive) food choices and less time and patience to read food labels and plan meals. So try to schedule a shopping trip in the early morning if it's on a weekend and avoid the after-dinner rush when most people shop.

When possible, leave the kids at home
Raise your hand if you ended up buying more than you intended when you went grocery shopping with your kids! It's difficult to devote time to food selection when you have to focus on appeasing your kids at the same time. There's no easy way to shop with children, so if possible, leave the little loved ones at home whenever possible for a more enjoyable (and cheaper) experience.

Using Organic Foods

While they are often more expensive, we do recommend women with PCOS eat organic foods whenever possible. Pesticides, hormones, and antibiotics (all of which can be found in nonorganic foods) may affect the health of women with PCOS, fertility in particular. We recommend choosing organic poultry, eggs, and grass-fed beef first and foremost. One exception to note is for seafood, as currently there are no government standards for what makes fish or shellfish organic. As such, we recommend looking for wild varieties of fish and seafood to reduce mercury exposure.

As of late, numerous studies have linked pesticides to developmental issues in children, cancer, and endocrine and reproductive problems, including infertility. To minimize your intake of pesticides, we recommend buying organic produce as much as possible, or at the very least for the fruits and vegetables listed on the Environmental Working Group's dirty dozen list of the most pesticide-laden produce in the U.S (see below), which ranks the order of the 12 highest pesticide-containing produce. Organic or not, wash all produce well by soaking, scrubbing, and rinsing under running water. Also, we encourage you to enjoy plenty of produce from the Clean 15 list (see below), which were found to contain the least amount of pesticides because of their protective outer skins.

By purchasing organic foods, you are also ensuring that the majority of the food you eat doesn't contain genetically modified organisms, commonly referred to as GMOs. Currently, we feel there's not enough evidence to show the safety in eating GMOs and their potential effects on human health. Some studies have shown that GMOs have the potential to cause serious health risks, including endocrine disruptions. Even still, the majority of the food in the United States is genetically modified. The most common sources are baby formula, corn (and all corn derivatives such as corn syrup), soy, cottonseed oil, canola oil, and sugar. The U.S. government doesn't require labeling of GMOs so it's impossible to tell which foods have GMOs in them, unless they are marked "Non-GMO" or are labeled 100% organic.

If you'd like more information on how to eat GMO-free, visit the Non-GMO Project (**nongmoproject.org**), which provides a database of verified GMO-free retailers and restaurants.

Storing Produce

Store these foods in the refrigerator:

Apples
Artichokes
Asparagus
Beans
Berries
Broccoli
Brussels Sprouts
Carrots
Cauliflower
Celery
Cherries
Corn
Cucumber
Eggplant
Fresh herbs (except basil)
Grapes
Green beans
Green onions
Leafy greens
Mushrooms
Okra
Peppers
Sprouts
Yellow squash
Zucchini

Store these foods at room temperature:

Acorn squash
Apricots
Avocados
Bananas
Basil (in water)
Butternut squash
Figs
Garlic
Ginger
Kiwi
Mangoes
Melons
Onions
Papayas
Peaches
Pears
Pineapple
Plums
Pomegranates
Potatoes
Spaghetti Squash
Tomato

Dirty Dozen

1. Apples
2. Strawberries
3. Grapes
4. Celery
5. Peaches
6. Spinach
7. Sweet bell peppers
8. Nectarines, imported
9. Cucumbers
10. Cherry tomatoes
11. Snap peas, imported
12. Potatoes

Clean 15

1. Avocados
2. Sweet corn
3. Pineapples
4. Cabbage
5. Sweet peas, frozen
6. Onions
7. Asparagus
8. Mangoes
9. Papayas
10. Kiwis
11. Eggplant
12. Grapefruit
13. Cantaloupe
14. Cauliflower
15. Sweet potatoes

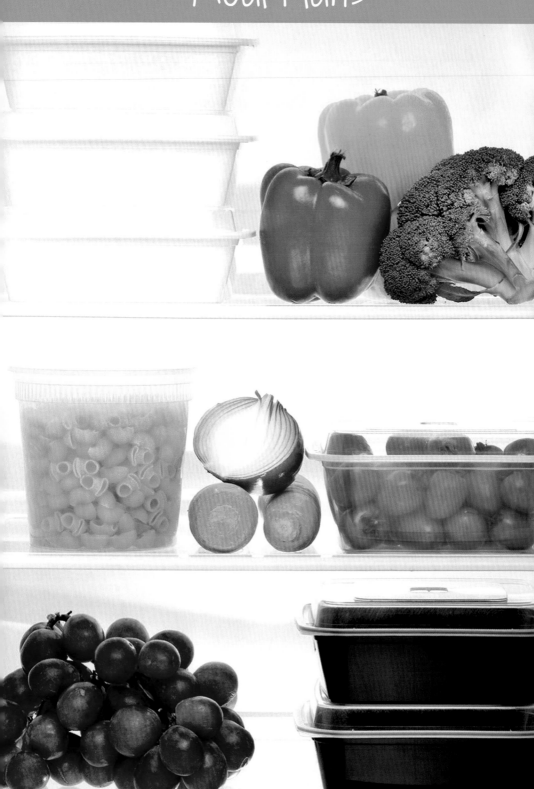

About the meal plans

These meal plans feature a variety of recipes used in this cookbook, which contain foods available at most supermarkets. These meal plans and recipes are low in sugar, sodium, and saturated fat and don't contain any artificial ingredients or trans fats. The majority of the protein is provided from eggs, fish, seafood, nuts, and poultry. Lean sources of red meat and soy products are included but in limited amounts. Dairy is limited to two or fewer servings each day. We've included plenty of slow carbohydrates to satisfy you, including whole grains, fruits, and vegetables.

Each day's menu generally averages between 1,600 to 1,800 calories and has less than 50% of calories coming from carbohydrates. Depending on your size, fitness level, genetics, and other unique concerns, this may or may not be enough to meet your personal needs. Always trust your body to determine whether you need to adjust these meal plans by adding more or less food. For specific nutrition advice, we recommend consulting with a registered dietitian nutritionist (RDN), such as the experts at the PCOS Nutrition Center, who can assess what's best for your nutritional needs.

Week One

Monday

Breakfast
Roasted Red Pepper and
    Pesto Egg Sandwich
1 cup strawberries

Snack
Coconut Almond Bar

Lunch
Mediterranean Chicken Wrap
1 cup grapes

Snack
Apple
2 tablespoons nut butter

Dinner
Broccoli and Cheddar
    Crustless Quiche
Field Greens Salad with
    Lemon Dijon Vinaigrette
Roasted Asparagus

Tuesday

Breakfast
Cherry Berry Smoothie

Snack
Coconut Almond Bar

Lunch
Broccoli and Cheddar
    Crustless Quiche
Orange

Snack
⅓ cup cashews
Peach

Dinner
Slow-Cooker Fire Roasted
    Tomato and White Bean Soup
Spinach Turkey Burger

Snack
1 ounce dark chocolate

Wednesday

Breakfast
Harvest Apple Oatmeal

Snack
Pear
2 tablespoons nut butter

Lunch
Italian Tuna Wrap
1 cup carrots
    and 2 tablespoons hummus
1 orange

Snack
Greek yogurt
1 cup strawberries
¼ cup low sugar granola

Dinner
Spicy Sesame Orange Chicken
    with Broccoli and Carrots
⅔ cup brown rice

Snack
½ cup pistachios

Thursday

Breakfast
Chocolate Peanut Butter Smoothie

Snack
⅓ cup dark chocolate
    covered almonds

Lunch
Wheat Berry Antipasti Salad
Orange

Snack
1 ounce cheese
8 whole grain crackers

Dinner
Grilled Salmon with
    Pineapple Mango Salsa
Corn on the Cobb with
Cilantro Lime Butter

Friday

Breakfast
Strawberry Coconut
    Breakfast Quinoa

Snack
Greek yogurt
1 cup raspberries

Lunch
Kale and Edamame Power
    Salad with Maple
    Almond Dressing
Pineapple Mango Salsa
15 corn tortilla chips

Snack
KIND Bar

Dinner
Cauliflower Crust Pizza
Nonno's Tomato Salad

Saturday

Breakfast
Banana Peanut Butter Pancakes

Snack
Tropical Green Smoothie

Lunch
Farro Minestrone Soup
Clementine

Snack
1 cup strawberries
⅓ cup pistachios

Dinner
Spaghetti Squash and Meatballs
Green Beans with Almonds

Snack
1 ounce dark chocolate

Sunday

Breakfast
California Veggie Omelet
2 slices sprouted grain bread
1 tablespoon butter

Lunch
Black Bean Cakes
Clementine

Snack
Single-serving pouch
    of tuna fish in water
6-8 whole grain crackers

Dinner
Sweet and Savory Roast Chicken
Tomato Lentil Vinaigrette Salad
Garlicky Spinach

Week Two

Monday

Breakfast
Maple Cinnamon Almond Smoothie

Snack
1 cup celery
2 tablespoons nut butter

Lunch
Farro Minestrone Soup
Grilled Chicken
    and Strawberry Spinach Salad

Snack
Apple
1 ounce cheese

Dinner
Japanese Eggplant and
    Mushroom Stir-Fry with Seitan

Tuesday

Breakfast
Canadian BLT Breakfast Sandwich

Snack
Kale and Apple Smoothie

Lunch
Ultimate Grilled
    Vegetable Sandwich
1/3 cup pistachios

Snack
Greek yogurt
1 cup strawberries

Dinner
Halibut with Walnut Pesto
Roasted Garlic Mashed
    Cauliflower
Tuscan Arugula Salad

Wednesday

Breakfast
Apple Crunch Yogurt Parfait

Snack
KIND Bar

Lunch
Asian Cobb Salad
1 slice sprouted grain bread
    with 1 teaspoon butter

Snack
1 tablespoon nut butter
Banana

Dinner
Spicy Cilantro Lime Chicken
2/3 cup wild rice
1/2 cup steamed broccoli

Thursday

Breakfast
Vanilla Blueberry Oatmeal

Snack
1/2 cup cottage cheese
1/4 cup walnuts
1 cup raspberries

Lunch
Mayo-less Chicken
    Salad Sandwich
1 cup strawberries

Snack
1 cup carrots
2 tablespoons hummus

Dinner
Salad Nicoise

Snack
3 cups air-popped popcorn

Friday

Breakfast
Berry Explosion Smoothie

Snack
Apple
2 tablespoons nut butter

Lunch
Tropical Tuna Chopped Salad
Pear

Snack
Greek yogurt
1/4 cup low sugar granola

Dinner
Slow-Cooker Vegetarian
    Black Bean Chili
Citrus Avocado Side Salad

Snack
1 ounce dark chocolate

Saturday

Breakfast
Huevos Rancheros

Snack
Tropical Green Smoothie

Lunch
Falafels with Cucumber Dill Sauce
Nonno's Tomato Salad

Snack
Peach
⅓ cup pistachios

Dinner
Sesame Ginger Glazed Salmon
Natalie's Cauliflower Fried "Rice"

Sunday

Breakfast
Italian Baked Eggs
1 slice sprouted grain bread

Lunch
Kale Cesar Salad with Shrimp
    and Chickpea Croutons
1 cup cherries

Snack
8 whole grain crackers
1 ounce cheese

Dinner
Savory Roast Turkey Breast
Garden Herb Quinoa,
    Chickpea, and Arugula Salad
Citrus-Glazed Carrots

Week Three

Monday

Breakfast
Slow-Cooker Pumpkin Pie
    Steel-Cut Oats

Snack
Coconut Almond Bar

Lunch
Five-Layer Turkey Sandwich
    with Cannellini Spread
Spinach Salad with Cinnamon
    Orange Vinaigrette

Snack
Banana
1 tablespoon nut butter

Dinner
Tempeh Teriyaki Stir-Fry

Tuesday

Breakfast
Chocolate Peanut Butter Smoothie

Snack
1 ounce cheese
8 whole grain crackers

Lunch
Egg Salad Sandwich
1 cup carrots
2 tablespoons hummus

Snack
1 cup blueberries
⅓ cup cashews

Dinner
Pork with Apples and Carrots
Garlic Roasted Cauliflower
Butter Lettuce with Apple
    Cider Vinaigrette

Wednesday

Breakfast
California Veggie Omelet
1 slice sprouted grain bread
1 cup strawberries

Snack
⅓ cup pistachios
Kiwi

Lunch
Edamame Veggie Burger
Citrus Avocado Salad

Snack
Greek yogurt
¼ cup low sugar granola

Dinner
Mediterranean Tuna Steaks
Barley Risotto
Roasted Asparagus

Snack
1 ounce dark chocolate

Thursday

Breakfast
Harvest Apple Oatmeal

Snack
Tropical Green Smoothie

Lunch
Vegetarian Taco Salad

Snack
½ cup low fat cottage cheese
1 cup blueberries

Dinner
Pineapple Chicken Kabobs

Snack
3 cups air-popped popcorn

Friday

Breakfast
Roasted Red Pepper
    and Pesto Egg Sandwich

Snack
Apple
2 tablespoons nut butter

Lunch
Super-Fast Soba Noodle Salad
Clementine

Snack
KIND bar

Dinner
Shrimp Tacos

Saturday

Breakfast
Coconut Almond Bar
1 cup strawberries

Snack
Greek yogurt
Mango

Lunch
Thai Style Coconut Shrimp Soup
Clementine

Snack
½ cup pistachios
1 cup cherries

Dinner
Marinated Flank Steak
Citrus-Glazed Carrots
Garlicky Spinach

Snack
1 ounce dark chocolate

Sunday

Breakfast
Buckwheat Pancakes
    with Blueberry Sauce

Snack
Coconut Almond Bar

Lunch
Moroccan Vegetable Stew
Orange

Snack
15 tortilla chips
¼ cup guacamole
½ cup salsa

Dinner
Slow-Cooker Stuffed Peppers
Parmesan Herb Spaghetti Squash

Week Four

Monday

Breakfast
Cherry Berry Smoothie

Snack
Coconut Almond Bar

Lunch
Moroccan Stew
Apple

Snack
1 ounce cheese
8 whole grain crackers

Dinner
Broccoli and Tempeh
   with Garlic Sauce

Snack
3 cups air-popped popcorn

Tuesday

Breakfast
Strawberry Coconut
   Breakfast Quinoa

Snack
Hard boiled egg
8 whole grain crackers

Lunch
Slow-Cooker Stuffed Peppers
Orange

Snack
Coconut Almond Bar

Dinner
Pecan-Crusted Trout
Sweet Potato Fries
Mini Kale Quiche

Wednesday

Breakfast
3 Mini Kale Quiches
1 cup strawberries

Snack
2 tablespoons nut butter
Celery sticks

Lunch
Mediterranean Chicken Wrap
1 cup cherries
1/3 cup pistachios

Snack
Greek yogurt
1/4 cup low sugar granola

Dinner
Shrimp Scampi with Broccoli

Thursday

Breakfast
Garden Frittata
Kiwi

Snack
Banana
2 tablespoons nut butter

Lunch
Peanut Noodles with Tofu and
Broccoli

Snack
3 cups air-popped popcorn

Dinner
Lemon Thyme Chicken
Quinoa with Peppers,
   Walnuts and Goat Cheese

Friday

Breakfast
Vanilla Blueberry Oatmeal

Snack
Peach
2 Mini Kale Quiches

Lunch
Garden Frittata
Black Bean and Toasted Corn Salad

Snack
1/3 cup dark chocolate
covered almonds

Dinner
Cauliflower Crust Pizza
Field Greens Salad with
   Lemon Dijon Vinaigrette

Saturday

Breakfast
Canadian BLT Breakfast Sandwich

Snack
Coconut Almond Bar
1 cup strawberries

Lunch
Lentil Soup
6 whole grain crackers
1 tablespoon hummus

Snack
2 tablespoons nut butter
Apple

Dinner
Polenta Casserole
Tuscan Arugula Salad

Sunday

Breakfast
Italian Baked Eggs
1 sprouted grain English muffin
Kiwi

Snack
1 cup carrots
2 tablespoons hummus

Lunch
Manhattan Clam Chowder
1 cup grapes

Snack
⅓ cup dark chocolate
    covered almonds

Dinner
Grilled Chicken Thighs
Corn on the Cobb with Cilantro
Lime Butter
Asian Slaw

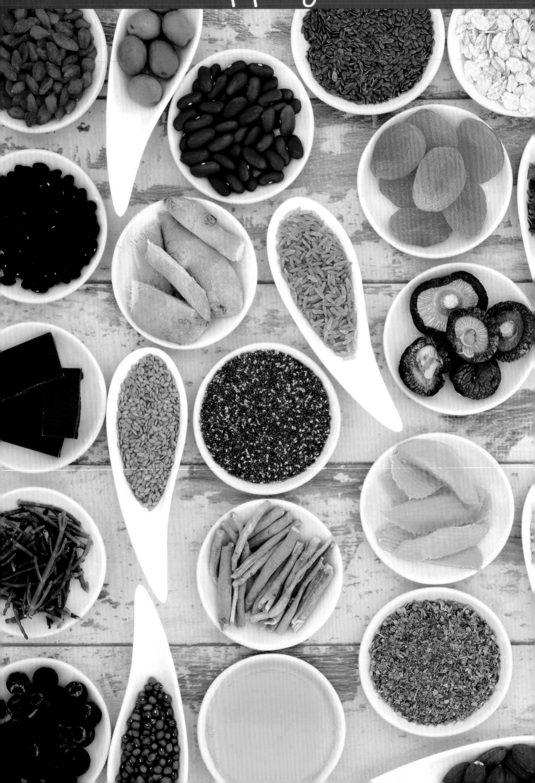

Pantry Staples

Kosher salt
Ground black pepper
Extra virgin olive oil
Cooking spray

Snacks

Strawberries
Grapes
Apples
Nut butter (almond, peanut
    butter, cashew)
Asparagus
Cashews
Pistachios
Peaches
Pears
Carrots
Raspberries
Oranges
Clementines
Hummus
Low sugar granola
Greek yogurt
Dark chocolate (at least 70%
    cocoa)
Dark chocolate covered almonds
Whole grain crackers
Tuna fish pouch
KIND bars

Roasted Red Pepper and Pesto Egg Sandwich

Egg
Provolone cheese (1 ounce)
Sprouted grain English muffins
Roasted red peppers
Pesto

No-Bake Coconut Almond Protein Bars

Rolled oats
Vanilla protein powder
Coconut flour
Almonds
Almond butter
Coconut oil
Honey
Pure vanilla extract
Unsweetened shredded coconut

Mediterranean Chicken Wrap

Whole wheat tortilla
    or sandwich wrap
Hummus
Cucumber (1)
Mixed greens
Grape tomatoes
Feta cheese
Red onion (1)
Chicken breast (4 ounces)
Kalamata olives

Broccoli and Cheddar Crustless Quiche

Canola oil
Onion (1)
Broccoli (1 head)
Extra sharp cheddar
    cheese (2 cups)
Quinoa flour
Eggs (6)
1% milk
Garlic powder
Kale (1 bunch)

Field Greens Salad with Lemon Dijon Vinaigrette

Mixed baby field greens
White wine vinegar
Lemon (1)
Dijon mustard
Honey

Cherry Berry Smoothie

Unsweetened vanilla coconut milk
Frozen dark sweet cherries (1 cup)
Blueberries (½ cup)
Chia seeds
Pure vanilla extract
Vanilla protein powder

Slow-Cooker Fire Roasted Tomato and White Bean Soup

1, (28 ounce) can fire roasted
    diced tomatoes
1, (15 ounce) can cannellini bean
1, (32 ounce) container low
    sodium vegetable broth
Brown rice
White onion (1)

Garlic
Dried basil
Bay leaves
Crushed red pepper
Swiss chard (3 cups)
Parmesan cheese (½ cup)

Spinach Turkey Burgers

93 to 95% lean ground
    turkey (1 pound)
Garlic
Spinach, frozen (¾ cup)
Lemon (1)
Eggs (1)
Whole wheat rolls (4)
Lettuce leaves
Tomato (1)
Red onion (1)

Harvest Apple Cinnamon Oatmeal

Unsweetened vanilla almond milk
Old fashioned oats
Chia seeds
Ground cinnamon
Slivered almonds
Pure vanilla extract
Granny Smith apple (1)

Italian-Style Tuna Salad Wrap

1, (5 ounce) can solid white tuna
Kalamata olives
Red bell pepper (1)
Green onion (1)
Sundried tomatoes
Fresh parsley
Lemon (1)
Arugula (½ cup)

Whole wheat sandwich wraps (2)

Spicy Orange Sesame Chicken with Broccoli and Carrots

Toasted sesame seeds
Orange (1)
Balsamic vinegar
Cornstarch
Garlic
Shallots
Red pepper flakes
Chicken breasts,
    boneless (1 pound)
Broccoli (1 head)
Carrots (5 large)
Brown rice

Chocolate Peanut Butter Banana Smoothie

Unsweetened coconut milk
Banana (1)
Peanut butter
Chocolate protein powder (such as
    Optimum Nutrition Whey Protein)
Ground cinnamon

Wheat Berry Antipasti Salad

Wheat berries (2 cups)
Grape tomatoes (1 cup)
Roasted Red Peppers
Mini fresh mozzarella balls (¾ cup)
1, (6 ounce) jar marinated
    artichoke hearts
Fresh basil
Balsamic vinegar
Honey
Arugula (6 cups)

Grilled Salmon with Pineapple Mango Salsa

Skinless salmon fillets (4)
Mango (1)
Pineapple (1)
Red onion (1)
Lime (1)
Cilantro
Red pepper
Good quality extra virgin olive oil

Corn on the Cobb with Cilantro Lime Butter

Corn, 4 ears
Unsalted butter (4 tablespoons)
Cilantro
Lime (1)

Strawberry Coconut Breakfast Quinoa

Quinoa (1 cup)
Unsweetened vanilla almond milk
Maple almond butter
    (such as Justin's)
Unsweetened shredded coconut
100% pure maple syrup
Strawberries (2 cups)

Kale and Edamame Power Salad with Maple Almond Dressing

Maple almond butter
Apple cider vinegar (⅓ cup)
100% maple syrup
Ground ginger
Garlic powder
Kale (8 cups)
Edamame, frozen shelled (1 cup)

Shredded carrots (1 cup)
Red bell pepper (1)
Red onion (1)
Avocado (1)
Zucchini (1)
Slivered almonds
Dried cranberries
Tortilla chips

Cauliflower Crust Pizza

Cauliflower (1 head)
Almond flour
Shredded cheddar cheese
    (⅓ cup)
Parmesan cheese
    (1 tablespoon)
Dried oregano
Dried basil
Garlic powder
Eggs (2)
Canola oil
Kale (2 cups)
Crushed red pepper
Pizza sauce (1 cup)
Shredded mozzarella cheese
    (4 ounces)
Beefsteak tomatoes (2)
Green pepper (1)
Good quality extra virgin olive oil
Red wine vinegar

Tropical Green Smoothie

Kefir, plain (¾ cup)
Kale (1 ½ cups)
Frozen raspberries (½ cup)
Frozen mango (½ cup)
Lite coconut milk (¼ cup)
Matcha (1 teaspoon)

Banana Peanut Butter Pancakes

Bananas (2)
Eggs (2)
Powdered Peanut Butter
Coconut flour
Unsweetened vanilla almond milk
Pure vanilla extract
Ground cinnamon
Coconut oil

Farro Minestrone Soup

Farro (1 cup)
Yellow onion (1)
Carrots (2 cups)
Celery (2)
Garlic
1, (32 ounce) can diced tomatoes
    (or 4 cups of chopped fresh
    tomatoes)
Dried Italian seasoning
1, (32 ounce) container
    low-sodium vegetable stock
1, (15.5 ounce) can kidney beans
1, (15.5 ounce) can garbanzo beans
Parmesan cheese (¾ cup)

Spaghetti Squash and Meatballs

Spaghetti squash (1 large)
Marinara sauce (4 cups)
Basil leaves
93% lean ground beef (1 pound)
½ pound ground chicken
Whole wheat panko
    bread crumbs (¾ cup)
Eggs (2)
Garlic powder

Fennel seed
Fresh parsley

Fresh thyme
Garlic

Green Beans with Almonds
Green beans (1 pound)
Good quality extra virgin olive oil
Garlic
Slivered almonds

California Veggie Omelet
Shiitake mushrooms ($\frac{1}{2}$ cup)
Green onion (1)
Tomato (1)
Spinach ($\frac{1}{2}$ cup)
Eggs (2)
Chives
Sprouted grain bread

Black Bean Cakes
Yellow onion (1)
Garlic
Red pepper (1)
Cumin
Coriander
1, (15.5 ounce) can black beans
Eggs (2)
Green onions (1)
Whole wheat panko ($\frac{1}{2}$ cup)
Cilantro
Sour cream (4 tablespoons)

Sweet and Savory Roast Chicken
1 whole chicken (3 pounds,
    bone included)
Red seedless grapes (1 pound)
Red onions (2)
Fresh rosemary

Tomato and Lentil Vinaigrette Salad
Lentils, dried (1 $\frac{1}{4}$ cup)
Carrots (1)
Onion (1)
Garlic
Bay leaf
Red wine vinegar
Grape tomatoes (2 cups)
Fresh parsley

Sautéed Garlicky Spinach
Good quality extra virgin olive oil
Garlic
Red pepper flakes
Spinach (4 cups)

Week Two

Pantry Staples
Kosher salt
Ground black pepper
Extra virgin olive oil
Cooking spray

Snacks
Celery
Apples
Carrot
Bananas
Raspberries
Cheese
Pistachios
Strawberries
Pears
Cherries
KIND bars
Cottage cheese
Greek yogurt
Walnuts
Hummus
Nut butter (almond, peanut
    butter, cashew)
Popcorn, air-popped
Dark chocolate (at least 70%
    cocoa)

Maple Cinnamon Almond Smoothie
Unsweetened almond milk
Maple almond butter
Banana (1)
Pure vanilla extract
Ground cinnamon

Grilled Chicken and Strawberry Spinach Salad
Skinless chicken breasts,
    boneless (¾ pound)
Lemons (2)
Baby spinach (4 cups)
Strawberries (1 cup)
Avocado (1)
Red onion (1)
Slivered almonds
Mint leaves
Feta cheese (¼ cup)
Honey
Garlic powder

Japanese Eggplant and Mushroom Stir-Fry with Seitan
Brown rice
Japanese eggplants (3)
Garlic chili paste
Paprika
Mexican style chili powder
Canola oil
Garlic
Ginger, fresh
Scallions (2)
1, (3.5 ounce) container shiitake
    mushrooms
1, (8 ounce) container baby
Portobello mushrooms

1, (20 ounce) container
    cubed seitan
Bragg liquid amino acids
Balsamic vinegar

Canadian "BLT" Breakfast Sandwich
Canadian bacon (1 slice)
Egg (1)
Sprouted grain English muffin
Arugula
Tomato (1)

Kale and Apple Green Smoothie
Vanilla coconut milk
Kale (1 ½ cups)
Granny Smith apple
Chia seeds
Matcha (1 teaspoon)

Ultimate Vegetable Sandwich
Sourdough bread, 4 slices
Zucchini (1)
Squash (1)
Red pepper (1)
Red onion (1)
¼ teaspoon kosher salt
½ teaspoon freshly ground
    black pepper
4 slices sourdough bread
½ cup arugula
Mozzarella cheese, packed
    in water (6 ounces)
Pesto

Halibut with Walnut Pesto
2, (6 ounce) skinless halibut fillets
Walnuts (½ cup)
Garlic (6 cloves)
Sweet basil (3 cups)
Parmesan cheese (½ cup)

Roasted Garlic Mashed Cauliflower
Cauliflower (1 large head)
Garlic (6 cloves)
Cream cheese
Chives

Tuscan Arugula Salad
Arugula (4 cups)
Walnuts
Roma tomatoes (2)
Olives
Balsamic vinegar
Parmesan cheese (2 tablespoons)

Apple Crunch Yogurt Parfait
1, (6 ounce) container Greek yogurt,
    plain, low-fat
Granny Smith apple (1)
KIND Healthy Grains Maple Quinoa
Granola
Ground cinnamon

Asian Cobb Salad
Rice wine vinegar
Ginger, fresh
Bragg liquid amino acids
Peanut butter
Canola oil
Sesame oil
Honey

Garlic powder
Sesame seeds
Romaine lettuce (8 cups)
Rotisserie chicken, small
Carrots, shredded (1 ½ cups)
Cara cara or navel oranges (2)
Slivered almonds, unsalted
Avocado (1)
Eggs (2)
Cilantro
Green onions (2)

Spicy Cilantro Lime Chicken
Chicken breasts, boneless
 and skinless
(1 pound)
Limes (2)
Garlic (5 cloves)
Cumin
Chili powder
Lite mayonnaise,
 olive oil based (¼ cup)
Greek yogurt, non-fat (¼ cup)
Jalapeño (1)
Cilantro
Broccoli (1 head)
Wild rice

Vanilla Blueberry Walnut Oatmeal
Unsweetened vanilla almond milk
Old fashioned oats
Chia seeds
Ground cinnamon
Walnuts
Pure vanilla extract
Blueberries (1 ½ cups)

Mayo-Less Chicken Salad Sandwich
Rotisserie chicken, small
Greek yogurt, plain
Dijon mustard
Celery (1 stalk)
Scallion (1)
Parsley
Sprouted grain bread (4)
Romaine lettuce (small bunch)

Salade Nicoise
Fingerling potatoes (½ pound)
Red wine vinegar
Shallots
Parsley
Hericot verts (French-style green
 beans), (8 ounces)
Mixed baby greens (4 cups)
Cherry tomatoes (1 cup)
Kalamata olives
Radishes (2)
Eggs (2)
2, (4 ounce) cans tuna
 fish, drained
Basil
Scallion (1)
Lemon (1)
Dijon Mustard

Berry Explosion Smoothie
Unsweetened vanilla almond milk
Frozen mixed berries (1 ½ cups)
Matcha (1 teaspoon)
Honey
Hemp hearts

Tropical Tuna Chopped Salad

1, (5 ounce) can wild albacore tuna
Mango (1)
Red bell pepper (1)
Avocado (1)
Carrot, large (1)
Jalapeño (1)
Cilantro
Green onion (2)
Lime (1)
Romaine lettuce (1 head)

Slow-Cooker Vegetarian Black Bean Chili

1, (28 ounce) can fire roasted
   diced tomatoes
3, (19 ounce) cans black beans
Jalapeño (1)
Red bell pepper (1)
Red onion (1)
Sweet potato (1)
Lime (1)
Cocoa powder
Mexican chili powder
Smoked paprika
Cayenne pepper
Cilantro
Avocados (1)
Cheddar cheese, shredded (1 cup)

Citrus Avocado Side Salad

Red onion (1)
Baby kale (3 cups)
Brussels sprouts (2 cups)
Avocado (1)
Cara cara or navel oranges (1)

White wine vinegar
Honey
Feta cheese, crumbled (¼ cup)

Tropical Green Smoothie

Kefir, plain (3/4 cup)
Kale (1 ½ cups)
Frozen raspberries (½ cup)
Frozen mango (½ cup)
Lite coconut milk (¼ cup)
Matcha (1 teaspoon)

Huevos Rancheros

Eggs (2)
Corn tortillas (2)
Avocado (1)
Sour cream, lite (2 tablespoons)
Cilantro

Falafels with Cucumber Dill Sauce

1 (15.5 ounce) can of garbanzo
   beans (chickpeas)
Yellow onion (1)
Garlic
Egg (1)
Baking powder
Cumin
Ground coriander
Parsley
Lemon (1)
Fava bean flour
Canola oil
1, (6 ounce) container Greek
   yogurt, plain
Dill, fresh
Garlic
Cucumber

Nonno's Tomato Salad
Beefsteak tomatoes (2)
Red onion (1)
Green pepper (1)
Good extra virgin olive oil
Red wine vinegar

Sesame Ginger Glazed Salmon
Toasted sesame oil
Rice wine vinegar
Low sodium soy sauce
Orange
Ginger, fresh
2, (6 ounce) boneless, skinless
    salmon fillets
Toasted sesame seeds

Natalie's Cauliflower Fried "Rice"
Cauliflower (1 head)
Canola oil
Onion
Garlic
Ginger, fresh
Mushrooms (1 ½ cups)
Zucchini (1)
Shredded carrots (1 cup)
Low sodium soy sauce
Cashews, unsalted
Green onion (1)
Eggs (1)
Sesame oil

Italian Baked Eggs
Grape tomatoes (½ pint)
Red bell pepper (1)
Red onion

Garlic
Tomato sauce (½ cup)
Eggs (6)
Mozzarella cheese, shredded
    (¼ cup)
Pecorino cheese (2 tablespoons)
Sprouted grain bread

Kale Caesar Salad with Shrimp and Chickpea Croutons
Greek yogurt
Garlic
Lemon (1)
Mustard
Anchovy paste
Parmesan cheese (3 tablespoons)
1, (14 ounce) can garbanzo beans
Extra virgin olive oil, divided
Kale (8 cups)
Shrimp, peeled and divined
    (1 pound)
Parmesan cheese (3 tablespoons)

Savory Roast Turkey Breast
Half turkey breast, bone in and skin
on (4 pounds)
Rosemary
Thyme
Sage
Lemon (1)
Unsalted butter

Garden Herb Quinoa, Chickpea and Arugula Salad

Quinoa, dry
Canola oil
Onion
Cumin
Parsley, fresh
Mint, fresh
Basil, fresh
Lemon (1)
Green onions (2)
Golden raisins (⅓ cup)
Slivered almonds
Feta cheese, crumbled (½ cup)
1, (15 ounce) can chickpeas
Arugula (4 cups)

Citrus-Glazed Carrots

Carrots (1 pound)
Orange (1)
Unsalted butter
Honey
Rosemary

Pantry Staples
Kosher salt
Ground black pepper
Extra virgin olive oil
Cooking spray

Snacks
Banana
Strawberries
Blueberries
Oranges
Carrots
Clementines
Cherries
Hummus
Nut butter (peanut, almond, cashew)
Cashews
Pistachios
Kiwi
Mango
Cheese
Greek yogurts
Cottage cheese
Low-sugar granola
Whole grain crackers
Dark chocolate (at least 70% cocoa)
Popcorn, air-popped
KIND bars
Whole grain tortilla chips
Guacamole

Slow-Cooker Pumpkin Pie Steel-cut Oats
Cold pressed coconut oil
Steel-cut oats
1, (16 ounce can) pumpkin puree
Brown sugar
Unsweetened vanilla almond milk
Pumpkin pie spice

No-Bake Coconut Almond Protein Bars
Rolled oats
Vanilla protein powder
Coconut flour
Almonds
Almond butter
Coconut oil
Honey
Pure vanilla extract
Unsweetened shredded coconut

Five-Layer Turkey Sandwich with Cannellini Bean Spread
Whole wheat pocket-less pita (1)
Cucumber (1)
Turkey breast (3 ounces)
Arugula
Tomato
1, (15 ounce) can cannellini beans
Basil, fresh
Parsley, fresh
Lemon (1)

Spinach Salad with Cinnamon Orange Vinaigrette
Sunflower oil
Rice wine vinegar

Ground cinnamon
Orange (1)
Baby spinach (6 cups)
Hemp hearts (4 tablespoons)

Tempeh Teriyaki Stir-Fry

Coconut oil plus 1 teaspoon
Tempeh (8 ounces)
Broccoli (1 head)
Carrots (1 ½ cups)
Snow peas (1 cup)
Brown rice
Cashew halves
Low-sodium soy sauce
Honey
Ginger, fresh

Chocolate Peanut Butter Banana Smoothie

Unsweetened coconut milk
Banana (1)
Peanut butter
Chocolate protein powder
    (such as Optimum Nutrition
    Whey Protein)
Ground cinnamon

Egg Salad Sandwich

Eggs (3)
Mayonnaise (olive oil based)
Whole grain mustard
Yellow mustard
Chives
Sprouted grain bread, low sodium
Romaine lettuce leaves

Pork with Apples and Carrots

4 ½ boneless skinless pork loins
    (about ½ inch thick or
    4 ounces each)
Ground ginger
Ground sage
Unsalted butter
1 Apple (Pink Lady)
Carrots (5 small)

Butter Lettuce Salad with Apple Cider Vinaigrette

Butter lettuce (4 cups)
Granny Smith apple (1)
Walnut halves (⅓ cup)
Balsamic vinegar
Apple cider vinegar
Honey
Peanut oil

Roasted Garlic Mashed Cauliflower

Cauliflower (1 large head)
Garlic (6 cloves)
Cream cheese
Chives

California Veggie Omelet

Shiitake mushrooms (½ cup)
Green onion (1)
Tomato (1)
Spinach (½ cup)
Eggs (2)
Chives
Sprouted grain bread

Edamame Veggie Burgers

Canola oil
Shiitake mushrooms (2 cups)
Edamame, shelled frozen
Garlic
Walnuts, chopped (¾ cup)
Parsley, fresh
Egg (1)
Low sodium soy sauce
Ginger, fresh
Cumin
Whole wheat panko
    bread crumbs (¼ cup)

Citrus Avocado Side Salad

Red onion (1)
Baby kale leaves (3 cups)
Brussels sprouts (2 cups)
Avocado (1)
Cara cara or navel oranges (2)
White wine vinegar
Honey
Feta cheese, crumbled (¼ cup)

Mediterranean Tuna Steaks

Lemon (1)
Garlic
Parsley, fresh
Basil, fresh
3 tuna steaks (4 ounces each)

Roasted Asparagus

Asparagus spears (1 pound)
Garlic (3 cloves)

Mushroom and Barley Risotto

Low sodium vegetable broth
    (3 cups)
Barley, quick cooking (1 cup)
Canola oil
White onion (1)
Garlic
Baby portabella mushrooms
    (1 ½ cups)
White wine
Lemon (1)
Parmesan cheese
    (2 tablespoons)
Parsley, fresh

Harvest Apple Cinnamon Oatmeal

Unsweetened vanilla almond milk
Old fashioned oats
Chia seeds
Ground cinnamon
Slivered almonds
Pure vanilla extract
Granny Smith apple (1)

Tropical Green Smoothie

Kefir, plain (¾ cup)
Kale (1 ½ cups)
Frozen raspberries (½ cup)
Frozen mango (½ cup)
Lite coconut milk (¼ cup)
Matcha (1 teaspoon)

Vegetarian Taco Salad with Creamy Cilantro Lime Dressing

Mixed field greens (4 cups)
Canola oil
Red onion (1)
Jalapeño pepper (1)
Pinto beans, canned (1 cup)
Mexican chili powder
Cumin
Garlic powder
Red bell pepper (1)
Grape tomatoes (½ cup)
Avocado (1)
Picante salsa
Cheddar cheese, shredded
    (¼ cup)
Greek yogurt
Lime (1)
Cilantro
Scallion (1)
12 whole grain, unsalted
    tortilla chips

Pineapple Chicken Kabobs

Extra virgin olive oil
Garlic
Lemon (1)
Parsley, fresh
Chicken breast, boneless, skinless
    (1 pound)
Pineapple (1)
Red bell pepper (1)
Red onion, cut into 1 to inch pieces
Squash (1)
Wild rice

Roasted Red Pepper and Pesto Egg Sandwich

Egg
Provolone cheese (1 ounce)
Sprouted grain English muffins
Roasted red peppers
Pesto

Super-Fast Soba Noodle Salad

1, (8 ounce) package buckwheat
    soba noodles
Cucumbers (2)
Red cabbage, shredded (2 cups)
Green onions (2)
Edamame, frozen, shelled
    (1 ½ cups)
Sesame seeds (¼ cup)
Cilantro
Sesame oil
Low sodium soy sauce
Balsamic vinegar
Pure maple syrup

Shrimp Tacos

Shrimp, peeled and deveined,
    large (1 pound)
Chili powder
Ground cumin
Pineapple (1)
Cabbage, shredded (3 cups)
Carrots, shredded (⅓ cup)
Avocado (1)
Cilantro
Limes (2)
12 corn tortillas

Thai-Style Coconut Shrimp Soup

1, (16 ounce) bag frozen shrimp (tail-on)
Canola oil
Garlic (4 cloves)
Ginger, fresh
Crushed red pepper
Low sodium vegetable broth (4 cups)
1, (13.5 ounce) can lite coconut milk
Oyster sauce
Low sodium soy sauce
Toasted sesame oil
(7 ounces) buckwheat soba noodles
Shiitake mushrooms (2 cups)
Baby bok choy (4 heads)
Cilantro
Scallions
Red chili pepper (1)
Lime (1)

Marinated Flank Steak

Flank steak, trimmed (1 ½ pounds)
Rosemary (fresh or dried)
Marjoram (fresh or dried)
Oregano (fresh or dried)
Crushed red pepper
Smoked paprika
Garlic (3 cloves)

Sautéed Garlicky Spinach

Good quality extra virgin olive oil
Garlic
Red pepper flakes
Spinach (5 ounces)

Citrus-Glazed Carrots

Carrots (1 pound)
Orange (1)
Unsalted butter
Honey
Rosemary, fresh

Buckwheat Lemon Blueberry Pancakes with Blueberry Sauce

Buckwheat flour
Almond flour
Coconut flour
Baking powder
Cornstarch
Chia seeds
Unsweetened almond milk
Egg (1)
Pure vanilla extract
Lemon (1)
Honey
Blueberries (1 cup)
Pure maple syrup
Unsweetened applesauce (½ cup)

Moroccan Vegetable Stew

Saffron (1 pinch)
Cumin
Ground ginger
Turmeric
Ground cinnamon
Cardamom
Coriander
Ground nutmeg
Extra virgin olive oil
Onion (1)
Garlic
Carrots (3)

Potato (1 small)
Sweet potato (1)
1, (28 ounce) can plum tomatoes
Quinoa
Cauliflower (1 head)
Zucchini (1)
Chickpeas, canned (1 cup)
Golden raisins (2 tablespoons)

Slow-Cooker Stuffed Peppers
Red peppers (5)
Cauliflower florets (2 heads)
Italian-Style chicken sausage
    (1 pound)
Marinara sauce (½ cup)
Walnuts, chopped (½ cup)
Parmesan cheese (½ cup)
Egg (1)
Whole wheat panko
    bread crumbs

Parmesan Herb Spaghetti Squash
Spaghetti squash (1)
Parsley, fresh
Parmesan cheese (2 tablespoons)

Pantry Staples
Kosher salt
Ground black pepper
Extra virgin olive oil
Cooking spray

Snacks
Apples
Kiwis
Bananas
Cherries
Peaches
Celery
Carrots
Cheese
Popcorn, air-popped
Whole grain crackers
Nut butter (peanut, almond, cashew)
Hummus
Greek yogurts
Low sugar granola
Dark chocolate covered almonds

Cherry Berry Smoothie
Unsweetened vanilla coconut milk
Dark sweet cherries, frozen
Blueberries (½ cup)
Chia seeds
Pure vanilla extract
Vanilla protein powder

No-Bake Coconut Almond Protein Bars
Rolled oats
Vanilla protein powder
Coconut flour
Almonds
Almond butter
Coconut oil
Honey
Pure vanilla extract
Unsweetened shredded coconut

Broccoli and Tempeh with Garlic Sauce
Brown rice
Garlic
Ginger, fresh
Chili garlic sauce
Low sodium soy sauce
Low sodium vegetable broth
Pure maple syrup
1, (8 ounce) package tempeh
Broccoli (1 head)
Asparagus (1 cup)
Cornstarch

Strawberry Coconut Breakfast Quinoa

Quinoa (1 cup)
Unsweetened vanilla almond milk
Maple almond butter
    (such as Justin's)
Unsweetened shredded coconut
100% pure maple syrup
Strawberries (2 cups)

Pecan-Crusted Trout

Pecans (½ cup)
Unsweetened shredded coconut
2, (6 ounce) trout fillets (skin intact)
Lemon (1)

Oven Sweet Potato "Fries"

Sweet potatoes (4)
Extra virgin olive oil
Garlic powder

Mini Quinoa Kale Quiches

Quinoa
Kale (1 bunch)
Mushrooms (1 cup)
Onion (1)
Garlic
Eggs (4)

Mediterranean Chicken Wrap

Whole wheat tortilla
    or sandwich wrap
Hummus
Cucumber (1)
Mixed greens
Grape tomatoes

Feta cheese
Red onion (1)
Chicken breast, 4 ounces
Kalamata olives

Shrimp Scampi with Broccoli

Whole wheat fettuccini pasta
    (1 pound)
Broccoli florets (2 heads)
Unsalted butter
Good quality extra virgin olive oil
Garlic (4 cloves)
Shrimp, cleaned with peel on
    (1 pound)
White wine
Lemon (1)
Red pepper flakes

Garden Frittata

Extra virgin olive oil
Asparagus (2 cups)
Red potatoes (3)
Shallot (1)
Eggs (8)
Low-fat milk (½ cup)
Tomato
Ricotta salata cheese (¼ cup)
Parsley, fresh
Chives

Peanut Noodles with Tofu and Broccoli

Low sodium soy sauce
1, (14 ounce) package
    extra firm tofu
1, (6 ounce) package soba noodles
(two wrapped bundles)

Garlic
Ginger, fresh
Honey
Peanut butter
Sesame oil
Broccoli florets, frozen (4 cups)
Cilantro
Scallions (2)
Unsalted peanuts, dry roasted
    (¼ cup)

Lemon Thyme
Baked Chicken Breasts
Chicken breasts, skinless
    (1 ½ pounds)
Lemon (1)
Garlic (6 cloves)
Thyme (6-8 springs)

Quinoa with Peppers,
Walnuts and Goat Cheese
Quinoa
Yellow pepper (1)
Orange pepper (1)
Walnuts, chopped (⅓ cup)
Lite raspberry vinaigrette dressing
    (such as Annie's Naturals)
Goat cheese (2 tablespoons)

Vanilla Blueberry
Walnut Oatmeal
Unsweetened vanilla almond milk
Old fashioned oats
Chia seeds
Ground cinnamon
Walnuts
Pure vanilla extract
Blueberries (1 ½ cups)

Black Bean and
Toasted Corn Salad
Corn, frozen (1 cup)
1, (15 ounce) can black beans
Red bell pepper (1)
Avocado (1)
Red onion (1)
Cilantro
Lime (1)
Ground cayenne pepper
Honey

Cauliflower Crust Pizza
Cauliflower (1 head)
Almond flour
Shredded cheddar cheese (⅓ cup)
Parmesan cheese (1 tablespoon)
Dried oregano
Dried basil
Garlic powder
Eggs (2)
Canola oil
Kale (2 cups)
Crushed red pepper
Pizza sauce (1 cup)
Shredded mozzarella cheese (4
ounces)
Beefsteak tomatoes (2)
Green pepper (1)
Good quality extra virgin olive oil
Red wine vinegar

Field Greens Salad
with Lemon Dijon
Vinaigrette
Mixed baby field greens
White wine vinegar
Lemon (1)

Dijon mustard
Honey

Canadian "BLT" Breakfast Sandwich
Canadian bacon (1 slice)
Egg (1)
Sprouted grain English muffin
Arugula
Tomato (1)

Vegetable Lentil Soup
Yellow onion (1)
Celery (2 stalks)
Carrots (1 ½ cups)
Garlic
Low-sodium vegetable broth
    (1 quart)
Lentils (1¼ cup lentils)
1, (15 ounce) can diced tomatoes
¼ teaspoon kosher salt
1 bay leaf
Kale (2 cups)

Italian Polenta Casserole
1, (18 ounce) package pre-cooked
    packaged polenta
White onion (1)
Garlic
Italian-Style chicken sausage
    links (3)
Zucchini (1)
1, (28 ounce) can fire roasted
    diced tomatoes
Spinach, frozen (1 ½ cups)
Crushed red pepper
Mozzarella cheese, part-skim
    (1 cup)

Tuscan Arugula Salad
Arugula (4 cups)
Walnuts
Roma tomatoes (2)
Olives
Balsamic vinegar
Parmesan cheese (2 tablespoons)

Italian Baked Eggs
Grape tomatoes (½ pint)
Red bell pepper (1)
Red onion (1)
Garlic
Tomato sauce (½ cup)
Eggs (6)
Mozzarella cheese, shredded
    (¼ cup)
Pecorino cheese (2 tablespoons)
Sprouted grain English muffin

Manhattan Clam Chowder
Canola oil
White onion (1)
Crushed red pepper
Garlic
Carrots (2 large)
Celery (3 stalks)
Baking potato (1)
Dry red wine
1, (28 ounce) can whole
    peeled tomatoes
Clam juice (1 cup)
Low sodium vegetable broth
    (4 cups)
Tomato paste
Bay leaves
Dried oregano
Clam meat, frozen (1 pound)

Parsley, fresh

Grilled Chicken Thighs
8 skinless, boneless chicken thighs
(about 2 pounds)
Dried parsley
Dried basil
Onion powder

Asian Slaw
1, (10 ounce) package shredded
     broccoli and carrot slaw
Cabbage, shredded (2 cups)
Green onions (4)
Sliced almonds (⅓ cup)
Sunflower seeds (½ cup)
Edamame, shelled (1 cup)
Rice wine vinegar
Low sodium soy sauce
Toasted sesame oil
Honey
Cilantro

Corn on the Cobb
with Cilantro Lime Butter
Corn, 4 ears
Unsalted butter (4 tablespoons)
Cilantro
Lime (1)

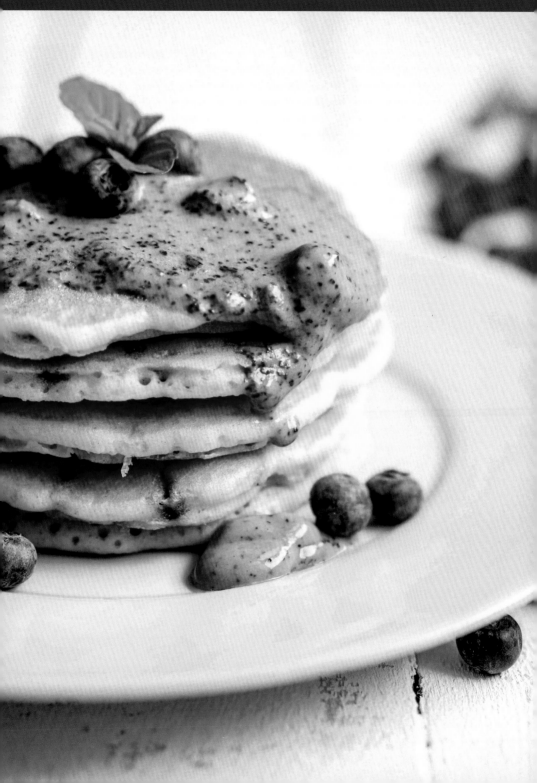

Slow-Cooker
Pumpkin Pie Steel-Cut Oats

Here's a tasty, heart healthy way to cook steel-cut oats while
you're asleep so they're ready for you in the morning.

Serves 4

Ingredients

- **1** tablespoon cold pressed coconut oil
- **1** cup steel-cut oats
- **2** cups (16 ounce can) pumpkin puree
- **1** tablespoon brown sugar
- **2** cups unsweetened vanilla almond milk
- **2** cups warm water
- ¼ teaspoon kosher salt
- **1 - 2** tablespoons pumpkin pie spice (according to taste)

Instructions

Melt coconut oil in a medium sauté pan. Add steel-cut oats and toast until lightly browned.

In a slow-cooker, combine pumpkin puree, sugar, almond milk, water, salt, and pumpkin pie spice. Mix well. Stir in oats. Set slow-cooker to low and cook 8 to 10 hours.

Tips

▸ Only use steel-cut oats. Other oats will burn or result in an undesired texture.
▸ This oatmeal can be portioned and stored in the refrigerator for up to 7 days. It reheats well in the microwave.
▸ Add chopped walnuts for added crunch.

270 calories • 40 g carbohydrate • 8 g fiber • 8 g fat (4 g saturated fat) • 8 g protein • 430 mg sodium

Mint and Matcha Power Smoothie

It's time to ditch your morning coffee for this tasty smoothie. Matcha is a concentrated green tea that's rich in antioxidants and shown to lower blood pressure and improve glucose levels.

Serves 1, 20 ounce smoothie

Ingredients

1 cup unsweetened almond milk

1 ½ cups baby spinach

2 tablespoons vanilla brown rice protein powder

1 teaspoon mint extract

1 teaspoon honey

1 teaspoon powdered matcha

2 cups ice cubes

Instructions

Combine all ingredients in blender. Blend on medium speed for 1 to 2 minutes.

Tips

► This recipe uses brown rice protein powder. You can use another variation, but make sure it contains little or no added sugar.

► Matcha can be purchased in natural-food stores and tea shops.

200 calories • 14 g carbohydrate • 4 g fiber • 3 g fat (0 g saturated fat) •19 g protein • 230 mg sodium

Maple Cinnamon Almond Smoothie

This smoothie is low in sugar and full of PCOS friendly ingredients. Almonds contain healthy monounsaturated fats, fiber, and antioxidants. Cinnamon is believed to aid against insulin resistance and may even help jump start menstrual cycles in women with PCOS.

Serves 1, 16 ounce smoothie

Ingredients

1 cup unsweetened almond milk
2 tablespoons maple almond butter
½ small banana (frozen)
½ teaspoon pure vanilla extract
1 teaspoon ground cinnamon
1 cup or **12** small ice cubes

Instructions

Combine all ingredients in blender. Blend on medium speed for 1 minute.

Tip

▸ Cut bananas in half and store them in the freezer to add to smoothies.

317 calories • 29 g carbohydrate • 7 g fiber • 17 g fat (1.5 g saturated fat) • 8 g protein • 181 mg sodium

Buckwheat Lemon Blueberry Pancakes with Blueberry Sauce

Most pancakes are full of carbohydrates and little nutritional value. This delicious version of a breakfast favorite is not only lower in carbohydrates, but contains heart healthy chia seeds and antioxidants.

Serves 4

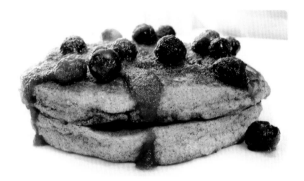

Ingredients

½ cup buckwheat flour
¼ cup almond flour
¼ cup coconut flour
1 tablespoon baking powder
2 tablespoons cornstarch
1 tablespoon chia seeds
¼ teaspoon salt
½ cup unsweetened
    almond milk
1 egg
1 teaspoon pure vanilla extract
Zest and juice of **1** lemon
1 teaspoon honey
½ cup water
1 cup blueberries, divided
1 tablespoon pure maple syrup
½ cup unsweetened
    applesauce
Cooking spray

Instructions

In a medium mixing bowl, whisk together flours, baking powder, cornstarch, chia seeds, and salt. Using a spoon, create a well in the center. Add almond milk, egg, lemon juice, zest, honey, and water. Mix well and set aside.

In a small sauce pan, combine ½ cup of blueberries, maple syrup, and applesauce. Heat over medium-high heat. Bring to a boil then reduce heat to a simmer, stirring continuously. Once blueberry sauce has reduced and thickened, set aside.

Instructions (cont.)

Fold remaining blueberries into pancake batter.

Spray a large skillet or griddle with cooking spray. Heat over medium-high heat. Once griddle is hot, drop ⅓ cup of batter on surface making silver dollar sized pancakes. Allow pancakes to cook 1 to 2 minutes on each side, turning when bubbles appear on edges. Continue with the rest of the batter.

Plate and serve with blueberry sauce.

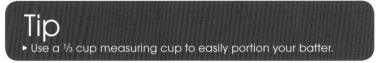

Tip

▸ Use a ⅓ cup measuring cup to easily portion your batter.

210 calories • 36 g carbohydrate • 6 g fiber • 5 g fat (1 g saturated fat) • 6 g protein • 550 mg sodium

Harvest Apple Cinnamon Oatmeal

Slow-cooked or old fashioned oats are whole grain and provide a good source of vicious fiber which is linked to a decreased risk of high cholesterol and diabetes. Chia seeds add to the fiber and along with almonds, provide healthy omega-3 fats in this delicious cinnamon apple oatmeal.

Serves 4

Ingredients

- **2 ½** cup unsweetened vanilla almond milk
- **2** cups old fashioned oats
- **1** tablespoon chia seeds
- **1** tablespoon ground cinnamon
- **⅓** cup slivered almonds
- **1** tablespoon pure vanilla extract
- **1** medium Granny Smith apple, chopped

Instructions

In a medium saucepan, heat almond milk over medium high heat for 2 to 3 minutes. Add oats, chia seeds, and cinnamon and stir to combine.

Reduce heat to low. Cook for 10 minutes, stirring occasionally.

Add almonds, vanilla, and apple. Stir to combine.

Tip

▸ For best flavor, use pure vanilla extract in this recipe.

218 calories • 30 g carbohydrate • 7 g fiber • 8 g fat (1 g saturated fat) • 7 g protein • 48 mg sodium

Italian Baked Eggs

This delicious, protein-rich dish will make everyone
think you spent lots of time in the kitchen.

Serves 4

Ingredients

½ pint grape tomatoes

1 red or orange bell pepper,
cored and cut into slices

¼ red onion, diced

2 cloves of garlic, roughly
chopped

2 tablespoons extra virgin
olive oil

⅛ teaspoon kosher salt

¼ teaspoon freshly ground
black pepper

½ cup tomato sauce

6 eggs

¼ cup mozzarella cheese,
shredded

2 tablespoons pecorino cheese

Instructions

Preheat oven to 475°F.

In a small baking dish, toss
grape tomatoes, pepper, onion,
and garlic with olive oil. Season
with salt and pepper. Bake in
oven for 15 minutes or until
tomatoes start to burst.

Remove vegetables from oven.
Pour tomato sauce into dish
and stir.

Pour eggs over top of the vegetable mixture. Top with mozzarella
cheese and return to oven. Bake
10 minutes or until whites are no
longer translucent.

Remove from oven and sprinkle
with pecorino cheese.

Serve immediately.

Tip

▸ To boost nutrient intake, add vegetables like spinach or kale
with eggs.

240 calories • 7 g carbohydrate • 2 g fiber • 13 g fat (4.5 g saturated fat) • 14 g protein • 240 mg sodium

Chocolate Peanut Butter Banana Smoothie

One of our most popular recipes from our Pinterest page, this delicious smoothie contains no added sugars and is rich in flavor. Enjoy it as a satisfying breakfast or snack. Cinnamon is believed to aid against insulin resistance and may even help jump start menstrual cycles in women with PCOS.

Serves 1, 16 ounce smoothie

Ingredients

- **1** cup of unsweetened coconut milk
- **1** small banana
- **2** tablespoons natural creamy peanut butter
- **1** scoop double rich chocolate protein powder (such as Optimum Nutrition Whey Protein)
- **½** teaspoon ground cinnamon
- **1** cup ice

Instructions

Place ingredients in a blender. Blend 2 to 3 minutes or until smooth.

Tip

▸ Unripe or slightly green bananas are lower in glycemic index than ripe ones.

465 calories • 34 g carbohydrate • 7 g fiber • 22 g fat (7 g saturated fat) • 32 g protein • 251 mg sodium

California Veggie Omelet

This omelet is filled with fresh veggies and provides high quality protein to start the day. Pair it with a side salad for a quick lunch or dinner.

Serves 1

Ingredients

1 teaspoon extra virgin olive oil
¼ cup diced fresh shiitake mushrooms
1 tablespoon finely chopped green onion
¼ cup diced tomato
½ cup chopped fresh spinach, packed
2 large eggs, beaten
⅛ teaspoon kosher salt
⅛ teaspoon freshly ground black pepper
1 teaspoon chives

Instructions

In a nonstick sauté pan, heat oil over medium heat. Cook mushrooms and onion until soft, about 5 minutes.

Add tomato and spinach and cook an additional 3 minutes. Mix in eggs, salt, and pepper. Cook until bottom and sides are firm, about 4 minutes (don't stir). Flip omelet in half and sprinkle with chives.

205 calories • 6 g carbohydrate • 2 g fiber • 14 g fat (4 g saturated fat) • 14 g protein • 453 mg sodium

No-Bake Coconut Almond Protein Bars

Here's an easy way to make your own protein bars at home.

Serves 6

Ingredients

⅓ cup rolled oats
⅓ cup vanilla protein powder
⅓ cup coconut flour
¼ cup almonds, diced
¼ teaspoon kosher salt
⅓ cup almond butter
2 tablespoons coconut oil
3 tablespoons honey
2 tablespoons pure
   vanilla extract
2 tablespoons unsweetened
   shredded coconut

Instructions

In a medium sized bowl, mix together oats, protein powder, coconut flour, almonds, and salt. Set aside.

Line a 9x9 inch baking dish with parchment paper. Set aside.

Heat a small sauce pan over medium heat. Add almond butter, coconut oil, honey, and vanilla. Heat until smooth, stirring continuously. Once all ingredients are melted, remove from heat.

Pour almond butter mixture into dry ingredients and mix well. Press mixture into baking dish. Sprinkle coconut over top and lightly press into mixture. Place dish in refrigerator and allow to set 3 hours.

Once bars are set, slice into 6 squares.

Tips

▶ Add cinnamon or cocoa powder to these bars for added antioxidants.
▶ Bars store best in refrigerator.

300 calories • 26 g carbohydrate • 3 g fiber • 17 g fat (6 g saturated fat) • 12 g protein • 240 mg sodium

Apple Crunch Yogurt Parfait

This breakfast is sure to get you started on the right foot in the morning. Traditional parfaits are typically high in sugar. Our version with plain yogurt and low sugar granola, leaves those added calories and carbohydrates behind without skimping on taste.

Serves 1

Ingredients

1, (6 ounce) container plain low fat Greek yogurt
½ medium Granny Smith apple, diced
¼ cup KIND Healthy Grains Maple Quinoa granola
½ teaspoon ground cinnamon

Instructions

In a 12 to 16 ounce glass or Mason jar, combine half of the apples and granola. Top with Greek yogurt. Layer remaining apple and granola. Sprinkle with cinnamon.

Tip
▸ Any variety of apples works well with this recipe.

270 calories • 39 g carbohydrate • 5 g fiber • 4 g fat (< 1 g saturated fat) • 21 g protein • 100 mg sodium

Huevos Rancheros

Here's a fast, heart-healthy way to use left-over
chili from last night's dinner for breakfast.

Serves 2

Ingredients

2 cups, leftover slow-cooker
vegetarian black bean chili
2 eggs
2 corn tortillas
½ avocado, sliced
2 tablespoons light sour cream
1 tablespoon cilantro,
roughly chopped

Instructions

In a medium sized sauté pan,
reheat chili over medium high
heat. Once chili starts to bubble,
crack eggs over top and cover
with lid. Cook approximately 5
minutes or until egg whites are
no longer translucent.

While the eggs are cooking,
heat tortillas according to package directions. Once heated,
place a tortilla on each dinner
plate.

When eggs are cooked, top each
tortilla with an egg and half of
the chili. Top with avocado, sour
cream, and cilantro.

Serve immediately.

330 calories • 32 g carbohydrate • 9 g fiber • 15 g fat (4 g saturated fat) • 18 g protein • 447 mg sodium

Canadian "BLT" Breakfast Sandwich

Substituting Canadian bacon for regular bacon
reduces the saturated fat in this breakfast favorite.

Serves 1

Ingredients

1 slice Canadian bacon
1 egg
⅛ teaspoon freshly ground
   black pepper
1 sprouted grain English
   muffin, toasted
4 - 5 baby arugula leaves
2 slices of tomato

Instructions

Heat a medium non-stick frying
pan over medium-high heat.
Add Canadian bacon. Cook
2 minutes and flip.

Move bacon to the side of the
pan. In the same frying pan, add
egg. Sprinkle egg with pepper.
Cook until whites are set then flip,
1 to 2 minutes.

Cook egg until desired doneness. Remove pan with egg
and Canadian bacon from heat.

On one side of English muffin,
add arugula leaves. Layer
with egg, bacon, tomato, and
remaining half of the muffin.

Serve immediately.

Tip

▶ This sandwich can be prepared on sprouted whole grain
   toast if you're not a fan of English muffins.

250 calories • 32 g carbohydrate • 6 g fiber • 8 g fat (2 g saturated fat) • 20 g protein • 570 mg sodium

Roasted Red Pepper and Pesto Egg Sandwich

Don't limit this tasty sandwich to breakfast alone-it's great for lunch or dinner.

Serves 1

Ingredients

1 teaspoon extra virgin olive oil
1 large egg, beaten
1 ounce provolone cheese
1 sprouted grain English muffin
3 slices roasted red peppers
2 teaspoons walnut pesto

(See Grilled Halibut and
Walnut Pesto recipe.)

Instructions

Heat oil in a medium non-stick skillet over medium heat. Add egg. Cook until edges are set. Add cheese and fold egg in half. Cook until egg is no longer runny.

Toast English muffin. Place egg on top of one half of English muffin. Top with roasted peppers. Spread pesto on remaining half of English muffin and place on top.

Tips

▸ Use jarred roasted red peppers to save time.
▸ If you don't have leftover pesto from the Grilled Halibut and Walnut Pesto recipe, use store bought.

454 calories • 35 g carbohydrate • 8 g fiber • 25 g fat (8 g saturated fat) • 23 g protein • 523 mg sodium

Vanilla Blueberry Walnut Oatmeal

Slow-cooked or old fashioned oats are whole grain and provide a good source of vicious fiber which is linked to a decreased risk of high cholesterol and diabetes. Chia seeds add to the fiber and along with walnuts, provide a healthy dose of omega-3 fats to this warm blueberry oatmeal.

Serves 4

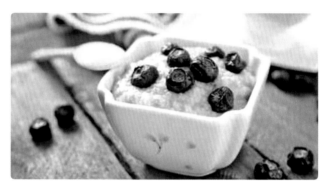

Ingredients

2 ½ cup unsweetened vanilla almond milk
2 cups old fashioned oats
1 tablespoon chia seeds
2 teaspoons ground cinnamon
⅓ cup chopped walnuts
1 tablespoon pure vanilla extract
1 ½ cup blueberries

Instructions

In a medium saucepan, heat almond milk over medium high heat for 2 to 3 minutes. Add oats, chia seeds and cinnamon and stir to combine. Reduce heat to low. Cook for 10 minutes, stirring occasionally.

Add walnuts, vanilla, and blueberries. Stir to combine.

Tips

▸ Use pure vanilla extract for this recipe. While expensive, it gives this dish its rich vanilla flavor.
▸ This oatmeal stores well in the refrigerator for leftovers.

238 calories • 32 g carbohydrate • 7 g fiber • 10 g fat (1 g saturated fat) • 7 g protein • 48 mg sodium

Cherry Berry Smoothie

Cherries are a low GI fruit that have been shown to fight inflammation.
Combined with blueberries, this smoothie is packed with antioxidants.

Makes 1, 20 ounce smoothie

Ingredients

1 cup unsweetened vanilla
   coconut milk
1 cup frozen dark sweet
   cherries, thawed
½ cup fresh blueberries
1 tablespoon chia seeds
½ teaspoon pure vanilla extract
1 scoop vanilla protein powder
   (such as RAW protein powder)
½ cup ice

Instructions

Place ingredients in blender.
Blend 2 to 3 minutes or until
smooth.

Tip

▸ It's important to blend well to mix up the protein powder.

315 calories • 40 g carbohydrate • 13 g fiber • 10 g fat (5 g saturated fat) • 22 g protein • 18 mg sodium

Strawberry Coconut Breakfast Quinoa

For a new go to hot cereal, try quinoa for breakfast. This versatile and high protein whole grain provides a satisfying meal in the morning. The combination of coconut, maple, and strawberries makes this a creamy sweet dish.

Serves 5 (makes 5 cups)

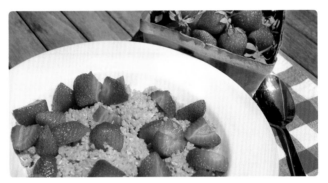

Ingredients

- **1** cup quinoa, dry
- **2** cups unsweetened vanilla almond milk
- **2** tablespoons maple almond butter (such as Justin's)
- **1** tablespoon unsweetened shredded coconut
- **1** tablespoon 100% pure maple syrup
- **2** cups sliced strawberries

Instructions

Place quinoa in a fine sieve or colander. Rinse well under running water, rubbing quinoa between hands for 1 minute; rinse and drain quinoa.

Place quinoa in a medium saucepan over medium heat. Stir constantly for 2 minutes to toast the quinoa. Stir in almond milk and bring to a slow boil over medium-high heat. Reduce heat to low and cover, stirring occasionally. Cook 15 to 20 minutes or until liquid has been absorbed. Remove from heat and fluff with fork.

While quinoa is warm, add almond butter, coconut, and maple syrup. Stir to combine. Stir in strawberries and serve warm.

Tips

- Rubbing the quinoa before cooking is important to remove its bitter outer coating.
- For a make-ahead breakfast, prepare quinoa (omitting strawberries) and store covered in a refrigerator for up to 4 days.
- When ready to eat, heat quinoa and top with strawberries.

237 calories • 34 g carbohydrate • 6 g fiber • 9 g fat (3 g saturated fat) • 7 g protein • 95 mg sodium

Berry Explosion Smoothie

Blueberries, strawberries, raspberries, and blackberries fill this smoothie with antioxidants. Hemp hearts are high in omega-3 fats and protein and are low in carbohydrates, making them a tasty option for women with PCOS.

Serves 1, 16 ounce smoothie

Ingredients

1 cup unsweetened vanilla almond milk

1 ½ cups frozen mixed berries (blueberries, strawberries, raspberries, blackberries)

1 teaspoon matcha

1 teaspoon honey

3 tablespoons hemp hearts

6 small ice cubes, or ¾ cup ice

Instructions

Place all ingredients in a blender. Blend for 1-2 minutes or desired texture.

Tips

▸ You can find frozen mixed berries in the freezer section of your supermarket. To freeze your own, rinse and hull berries, dry well, and store in a freezer bag.

▸ Matcha is a concentrated green tea powder that contains a small amount of caffeine. It's sold in many natural-food stores and tea shops.

300 calories • 29 g carbohydrate • 9 g fiber • 16 g fat (1.5 g saturated fat) • 12 g protein • 180 mg sodium

Kale and Apple Green Smoothie

Makes 1, 16 ounce smoothie

Ingredients

¾ cup vanilla coconut milk

1 ½ cups kale, chopped

1 green apple, chopped

1 tablespoon plus 1 teaspoon chia seeds

1 teaspoon matcha

½ cup ice

Instructions

Combine all ingredients in blender. Blend on medium speed for 1 to 2 minutes.

Tip

▸ Matcha is a concentrated form of green tea that contains caffeine. It's sold in powder form in most health stores or tea shops.

310 calories • 43 g carbohydrate • 14 g fiber • 13 g fat (4 g saturated fat) • 9 g protein • 60 mg sodium

Tropical Green Smoothie

This smoothie is sure to get you energized in the morning. It's full of antioxidants and provides a boost of caffeine from the matcha. Kefir is a drinking-style yogurt that contains beneficial probiotics.

Makes 1, 16 ounce smoothie

Ingredients

¾ cup plain kefir
1 ½ cups kale, chopped
½ cup frozen raspberries
½ cup frozen mango
¼ cup lite coconut milk
1 teaspoon matcha
½ cup ice

Instructions

Combine all ingredients in blender. Blend on medium speed for 1 to 2 minutes.

Tip

▸ Matcha is a concentrated form of green tea that contains caffeine. It's sold in powder form in most health stores or tea shops.

230 calories • 34 g carbohydrate • 9 g fiber • 6 g fat (1.5 g saturated fat) • 14 g protein • 135 mg sodium

Banana
Peanut Butter Pancakes

Here's a grain-less version of a breakfast classic
that's low in carbohydrates but full of flavor.

Serves 2

Ingredients

2 bananas, sliced
2 eggs
3 tablespoon powdered
   peanut butter
1 tablespoon coconut flour
3 tablespoons unsweetened
vanilla almond milk
1 teaspoon pure vanilla extract
½ teaspoon ground cinnamon
1 tablespoons coconut oil

Instructions

In a medium bowl combine bananas, eggs, peanut butter, coconut flour, almond milk, vanilla, and cinnamon. Mix well with a whisk or hand mixer, leaving some lumps in the batter.

Heat a skillet or griddle over medium-high heat. Add coconut oil.

Once griddle is hot, drop ½ cup of batter on surface. Allow pancakes to cook 1 to 2 minutes on each side, turning when bubbles appear on edges. Continue with the rest of the batter.

Tip
▸ Add strawberries or other fruit to make this taste like a peanut butter and jelly sandwich.

278 calories • 25 g carbohydrate • 4 g fiber • 15 g fat (9 g saturated fat) • 12 g protein • 174 mg sodium

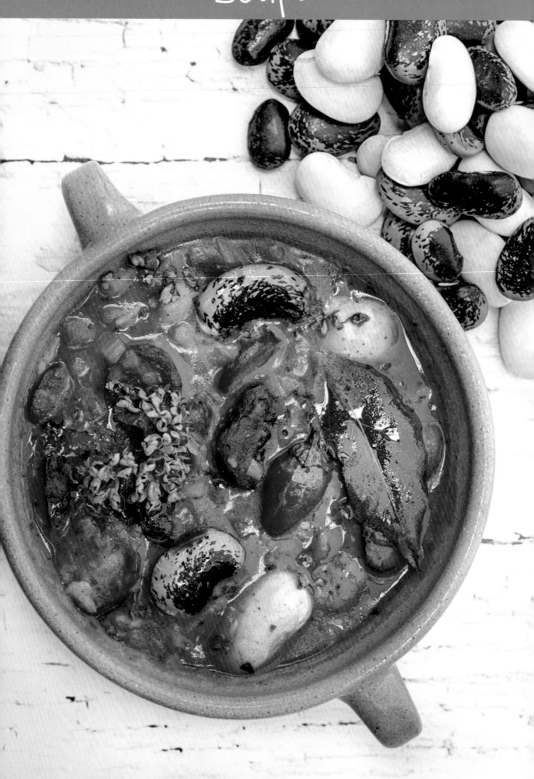

Slow-Cooker Fire Roasted Tomato and White Bean Soup

This soup is a nutrition power house. Swiss chard not only provides fiber and magnesium, it's also an excellent source of vitamins A, C, and K.

Serves 6

Ingredients

1, (28 ounce) can fire roasted diced tomatoes, undrained
1, (15 ounce) can cannellini beans, rinsed and drained
5 cups low sodium vegetable broth
½ cup brown rice, uncooked
¾ cup white onion, finely chopped
4 cloves garlic, minced
1 tablespoon dried basil
2 bay leaves
⅛ teaspoon crushed red pepper
¼ teaspoon salt
¼ teaspoon freshly ground black pepper
3 cups Swiss chard, chopped
½ cup shaved parmesan cheese

Instructions

Combine tomatoes, beans, broth, rice, onion, garlic, basil, bay leaves, red pepper, salt, and pepper in a 6 to 7 quart slow-cooker. Cook on low for 6 hours.

Add Swiss chard and cook 15 minutes or until leaves are tender. Discard bay leaves.

Serve in bowls and top with shaved parmesan cheese.

Tip

 This soup freezes well and can be used for meals later in the week.

200 calories • 30 g carbohydrate • 5 g fiber • 3 g fat (1.5 g saturated fat) • 11 g protein • 370 mg sodium

Manhattan Clam Chowder

Clams are an excellent source of iron. One serving of this soup provides over 100% of the recommended daily iron intake.

Serves 6

Ingredients

2 tablespoons canola oil
1 cup white onion, chopped
⅛ teaspoon crushed red pepper
3 cloves garlic, minced
2 large carrots or
  1 cup, chopped
3 celery stalks, chopped
1 large baking potato or
  1 ½ cups, peeled and
  cut in **½** inch cubes
¼ cup dry red wine
1, (28 ounce) can whole peeled
  tomatoes, undrained
1 cup clam juice
4 cups low sodium
  vegetable broth
3 tablespoons tomato paste
3 bay leaves
2 teaspoons dried oregano
¼ teaspoon freshly ground
  black pepper
1 pound frozen clam meat,
  unthawed
1 cup fresh Italian flat leaf
  parsley, roughly chopped

Instructions

In a 6 to 8 quart Dutch oven or sauce pan, heat oil over medium-high heat. Add onion and crushed red pepper. Cook until onion is translucent, about 3 to 5 minutes.

Add garlic, carrots, celery, and potatoes. Sauté vegetables for 5 minutes, stirring continuously. Scrape caramelized bits of onion and vegetables off pan. Add red wine. Reduce heat to medium.

Using kitchen shears roughly cut apart whole peeled tomatoes (while in can). Add tomatoes, clam juice, broth, tomato paste, bay leaves, oregano, and pepper. Cover and cook until vegetables are tender, stirring occasionally, about 25 to 30 minutes.

When vegetables are tender, increase heat to medium-high heat and stir in clams. Cook 3 minutes. Remove from heat and stir.

When vegetables are tender, increase heat to medium-high heat and stir in clams. Cook 3 minutes. Remove from heat and stir in fresh parsley. Serve immediately.

230 calories • 16 g carbohydrate • 2 g fiber • 6 g fat (2.5 g saturated fat) • 22 g protein • 350 mg sodium

Moroccan Vegetable Stew

This stew is full of spices and flavor. Cinnamon, ginger, and turmeric are believed to help in regulating blood sugar.

Serves 5

Ingredients

Spice mixture:

2 pinches of saffron
1 teaspoon cumin
1 teaspoon ground ginger
½ teaspoon kosher salt
½ teaspoon turmeric
½ teaspoon ground cinnamon
½ teaspoon cardamom
½ teaspoon coriander
½ teaspoon ground nutmeg
½ teaspoon freshly ground black pepper

Soup mixture:

2 tablespoons extra virgin olive oil
1 small onion, diced
3 garlic cloves, diced
3 carrots, peeled and sliced
1 small potato, peeled and sliced in quarters
½ sweet potato, peeled and sliced in quarters
1, (28 ounce) can plum tomatoes
1 cup quinoa
½ head of cauliflower, stemmed and cut into florets
1 small zucchini, sliced
1 cup canned chickpeas, rinsed and drained
2 tablespoons golden raisins

Instructions

Combine all spices in a small bowl and mix well. Heat a 5 to 6 quart Dutch oven or large sauce pan over medium-high heat. Add spice mixture and toast until fragrant, about 1 minute. Return toasted spices to small bowl and set aside.

In the same pan, heat oil over medium heat and add onions. Cook until softened, about 5 minutes. Add garlic, carrots, and potatoes. Sauté 2 to 3 minutes.

With tomatoes in can, cut into smaller pieces using kitchen shears. Add to pan. Next, stir in spices. Bring to a simmer and cook until vegetables are just tender, about 20 minutes.

While vegetables are cooking, cook quinoa according to package directions.

Once potatoes and carrots are just tender, add cauliflower, zucchini, and chickpeas. Cook until vegetables are tender, about 10 minutes. Stir in raisins.

Serve over ⅓ cup quinoa.

Tips

- Slice vegetables no more than ¼ inch thick to quicken cook time.
- Be sure to rinse and scrub quinoa prior to cooking to remove outer coating.

270 calories • 40 g carbohydrate • 10 g fiber • 10 g fat (1 g saturated fat) • 10 g protein • 420 mg sodium

Slow-Cooker Vegetarian Black Bean Chili

You won't miss the meat in this hearty vegetarian chili.
Each satisfying bowl packs plenty of flavor, fiber, and protein.

Serves 6

Ingredients

- 1, (28 ounce) can fire roasted diced tomatoes, undrained
- 3, (19 ounce) cans black beans, drained and rinsed
- 1 jalapeño, seeded and diced
- 1 red bell pepper,seeded and diced
- 1 red onion, diced
- 1 sweet potato, peeled and diced in ½ inch cubes
- Zest and juice of 1 lime
- 1 tablespoon cocoa powder
- 1 tablespoon Mexican chili powder
- 1 teaspoon smoked paprika
- ⅛ teaspoon cayenne pepper
- 1 teaspoon extra virgin olive oil
- 2 tablespoons cilantro leaves, roughly chopped
- 2 avocados, diced
- 1 cup shredded cheddar cheese

Instructions

Combine tomatoes, beans, jalapeño, pepper, onion, potato, lime zest and juice, cocoa powder, chili powder, paprika, cayenne pepper, and oil in a 6-7 quart slow-cooker. Mix well.

Cook on low for 7 ½ to 8 hours.

After chili has cooked, stir in cilantro leaves.

Divide in bowls and top each serving evenly with avocado and cheese.

Tips

- ▸ Cut your cooking time in half by setting your slow-cooker on the high setting.
- ▸ This chili freezes well for future meals.

300 calories • 31 g carbohydrate • 13 g fiber • 14 g fat (5 g saturated fat) • 13 g protein • 447 mg sodium

Thai-Style Coconut Shrimp Soup

Spicy foods are known to boost production of serotonin, a "feelgood" hormone. This one pot meal is packed with flavor! Shrimp and bok choy make it rich in calcium.

Serves 4

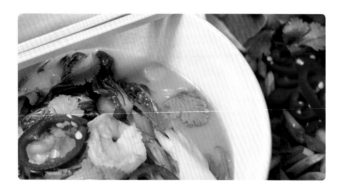

Ingredients

1, (16 ounce) bag frozen shrimp (tail-on), thawed

1 teaspoon canola oil

4 cloves garlic, minced

1 tablespoon fresh ginger, minced

1/8 teaspoon crushed red pepper

4 cups low sodium vegetable broth

1/2 cup water

1, (13.5 ounce) can lite coconut milk

2 teaspoons oyster sauce

2 teaspoons low sodium tamari or soy sauce

1 teaspoon toasted sesame oil

7 ounce buckwheat soba noodles

2 cups shiitake mushrooms, sliced

4 heads of baby bok choy, quartered

1/2 cup cilantro leaves

2 scallions, diced

1 red chili pepper, sliced in wheels (seeds removed)

1 lime, cut into wedges

Instructions

Rinse and drain shrimp. Set aside.

In a large Dutch oven or stock pot, heat canola oil over medium-high heat. Add garlic, ginger, and crushed red pepper. Cook until just fragrant, about 1 to 2 minutes.

Add vegetable broth, water, coconut milk, sweet chili sauce, tamari, oyster sauce, and sesame oil. Bring to a boil.

While broth is boiling, add soba noodles and mushrooms. Cook one minute. Add shrimp and bokchoy. Cook until shrimp turn pink, about 2 to 3 minutes. Remove from heat and garnish with cilantro leaves, scallions, chili pepper, and lime.

Serve immediately.

Tips

▸ For more spice, increase the crushed red pepper to ¼ teaspoon.
▸ A jalapeño pepper can be substituted for the red chili.

340 calories • 42 g carbohydrate • 3 g fiber • 10 g fat (< 1 g saturated fat) • 24 g protein • 525 mg sodium

Vegetable Lentil Soup

This hearty vegetarian soup is rich in iron, fiber, vitamins and minerals thanks to low GI lentils, tomatoes and kale.

Serves 6 (makes 6 cups)

Ingredients

- 1 tablespoon extra virgin olive oil
- ½ cup chopped medium yellow onion
- 2 celery stalks, chopped
- 1 ½ cup chopped carrots
- 3 garlic cloves, minced
- 1 quart low-sodium vegetable broth
- 1 ¼ cup lentils
- 15 ounce can diced tomatoes
- ¼ teaspoon kosher salt
- ½ teaspoon freshly ground pepper
- 1 teaspoon Italian seasoning
- 1 bay leaf
- 2 cups kale, chopped

Instructions

Heat oil in a large saucepan over medium heat, about 2 minutes. Add onions, celery, and carrots. Cook over medium heat, stirring occasionally until soft, about 8 to 10 minutes.

Stir in garlic. Add broth, lentils, tomatoes, salt, pepper, Italian seasoning, and bay leaf and stir. Bring to a boil.

Cover. Reduce heat to low and cook until lentils are soft, about 25 minutes. Remove bay leaf. Add kale and stir until wilted.

Serve immediately.

Tip

▶ To make this recipe even quicker, buy already chopped onions, carrots and celery.

144 calories • 20 g carbohydrate • 7 g fiber • 5 g fat (1 g saturated fat) • 6 g protein • 326 mg sodium

Farro Minestrone Soup

This hearty soup is perfect on a cold rainy day. Farro is a sturdy, ancient whole grain with a nutty flavor similar to brown rice. It's rich in fiber, magnesium and vitamins A, B, C, and E.

Serves 12 (makes 12 cups)

Ingredients

- **1** cup farro, uncooked
- **1** tablespoon extra virgin olive oil
- **1** cup chopped yellow onion
- **2** cups chopped carrots
- **1** cup chopped celery
- **3** cloves of garlic, sliced
- **32** ounce can of diced tomatoes (or 4 cups of chopped fresh tomatoes)
- **1** tablespoon dried Italian seasoning
- **1** teaspoon kosher salt
- **1** teaspoon freshly ground pepper
- **32** ounces of low-sodium vegetable stock
- **15.5** ounce can kidney beans, rinsed and drained
- **15.5** ounce can garbanzo (chickpeas) beans, rinsed and drained
- **¾** cup freshly grated parmesan cheese

Instructions

Cook farro according to package instructions. Fluff with fork. Set aside.

While farro is cooking, chop vegetables. In a large saucepan add oil, onions, carrots, celery, and garlic. Cook covered over low heat until softened, about 10 to 15 minutes, stirring occasionally.

Add tomatoes, Italian seasoning, salt, pepper, and stock. Cook covered over low to medium heat for 20 minutes, stirring occasionally.

Stir in kidney and garbanzo beans and farro. Cook covered for 10 minutes.

Top each serving with 1 tablespoon of parmesan cheese.

Tips

- ▸ Use quick-cooking farro to save time.
- ▸ Wheat berries or barley can be substituted for farro.

230 calories • 38 g carbohydrate • 10 g fiber • 4 g fat (1 g saturated fat) • 11 g protein • 404 mg sodium

Classic Chicken Noodle Soup

This homemade chicken noodle soup is a mix of fresh herbs, vegetables, and udon noodles. Just what the dietitian ordered!

Serves 8

Ingredients

1 tablespoon extra virgin olive oil
1 cup carrots, chopped
1 cup celery, chopped
1 yellow onion, chopped
5 cups chicken broth
3 cups water
1 package of fresh poultry herbs blend (rosemary, sage, and thyme)
Bakers twine
2 bay leaves
1 rotisserie chicken, skin removed and meat pulled from bone (approximately 4 cups)
½ teaspoon garlic powder
½ teaspoon kosher salt
½ teaspoon freshly ground black pepper
14 ounces plain udon noodles, broken into thirds
1 cup fresh parsley, roughly chopped
2 scallions, diced

Instructions

In a large stock pot or Dutch oven, heat olive oil over medium-high heat. Add carrots, celery, and onions. Sauté until onions are translucent, about 5 minutes. Once vegetables start to soften, add broth and water. Lower heat to medium.

Make a bundle out of poultry herbs and tie tightly with the baker's twine. Toss bundle and bay leaves into soup. Add chicken, garlic powder, salt, and pepper to soup. Cover, raise heat to high and allow soup to reach a boil. Once soup has reached a boil, bring to a simmer and cook 5 minutes or until vegetables are tender.

While soup is cooking, prepare udon noodles according to package directions. When noodles are cooked and drained, divide them among 8 bowls.

Remove soup from heat. Remove and discard herb bundle. Stir in parsley. Ladle soup over noodles and garnish with scallions. Serve immediately.

170 calories • 11 g carbohydrate • 1 g fiber • 4.5 g fat (1 g saturated fat) • 22 g protein • 370 mg sodium

Vegetable Red Curry with Tofu

This flavorful stew-like dish is quick and full of green veggies!

Serves 4

Ingredients

- **1** tablespoon canola oil
- **3** tablespoons Thai red curry paste
- **1** tablespoon fresh ginger, minced
- **1** cup diced onion
- **2** tablespoons minced garlic
- **1** cup low sodium vegetable broth
- **2**, (14 ounce) cans lite coconut milk
- **1** tablespoon brown sugar
- **1** tablespoon low sodium soy sauce
- **2** cups sugar snap peas
- **1** pound baby bok choy
- **2** cups asparagus, trimmed and cut in half
- **1**, (14 ounce) package extra firm tofu, pressed and cut into 1 inch cubes

Instructions

Heat canola oil in large deep sauce pan or Dutch oven over medium-high heat. Add red curry paste, ginger, onions, and garlic. Cook until fragrant.

Whisk in vegetable broth, coconut milk, brown sugar, and soy sauce. Bring to a boil.

Add snap peas, bok choy, and asparagus. Cover and cook 10 minutes. Once vegetables are just firm, add tofu. Cook 5 minutes.

Serve immediately.

Tips
- For a gluten-free meal, use tamari in place of soy sauce.
- Serve this dish over ⅓ cup cooked brown rice for a more substantial meal.

300 calories • 15 g carbohydrate • 4 g fiber • 19 g fat (9 g saturated fat) • 12 g protein • 370 mg sodium

Carrot Coriander Soup

A yummy soup for a cool evening! This recipe is shared by our friend Susan Adams, registered dietitian and Assistant Professor of Nutrition at LaSalle University.

Serves 8

Ingredients

1 large onion, sliced thin
2 tablespoons canola oil
1 garlic glove, minced
1 teaspoon ground coriander
10 carrots, fresh (about 1 ½ pounds), sliced thin
2 new potatoes (medium size), peeled and quartered
5 cups rich low sodium chicken broth
1 ¼ cups freshly squeezed orange juice
½ teaspoon kosher salt
½ teaspoon white pepper
¼ cup minced fresh cilantro (for garnish)

Instructions

Place onion and oil in a large stock pot. Cook over medium low heat, stirring until the onion is softened. Add garlic and cook the mixture, stirring constantly, for 2 minutes.

Add coriander and cook the mixture for 2 more minutes, continuing to stir. Add the carrots and potatoes and cook the mixture, still stirring, for 2 minutes longer. Add stock, juice, salt and white pepper. Bring the liquid to a boil, cover and lower the heat to a simmer. Continue to cook the mixture for 20 to 30 minutes on low heat, until the carrots are tender, stirring occasionally.

Carefully puree the soup in batches in a blender. Pour soup into bowls. Garnish with fresh cilantro.

Serve hot.

Tips

► Hold down the lid of the blender with a kitchen towel.
► A dollop of sour cream is delicious as a garnish.
► Store leftover soup covered in the refrigerator for up to 3 days or freeze up to 3 months.

143 calories • 24 g carbohydrate • 4 g fiber • 4 g fat (< 1 g saturated fat) • 4 g protein • 565 mg sodium

Salads

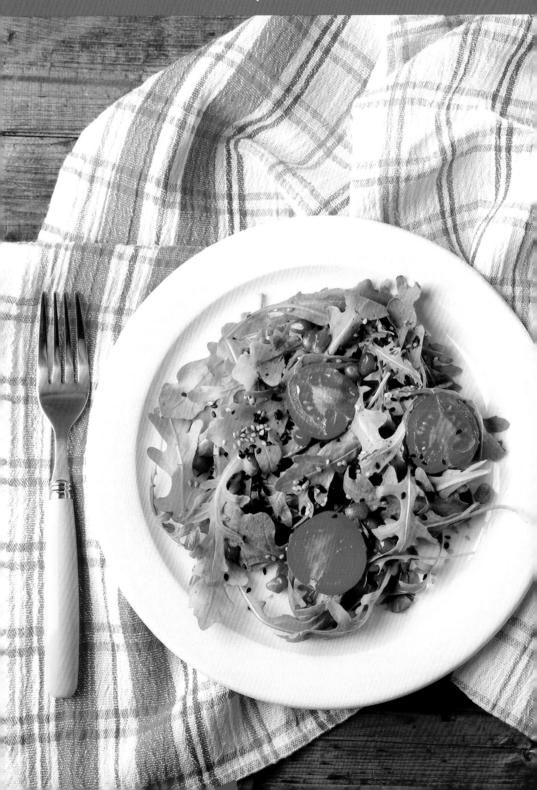

Grilled Chicken and Strawberry Spinach Salad

This delicious salad is full of vitamin C, iron, and healthy fats.

Serves 2

Ingredients

- ¾ pound of boneless, skinless chicken breast
- **2** tablespoons extra virgin olive oil, divided
- Juice of **2** lemons, divided
- ¼ teaspoon kosher salt
- ¼ teaspoon freshly ground black pepper
- **4** cups baby spinach, washed
- **1** cup strawberries, sliced
- ¼ cup avocado, diced
- ¼ cup sliced red onion
- **2** tablespoons slivered almonds
- **2** tablespoons mint leaves, roughly chopped
- ¼ cup feta cheese
- ½ teaspoon honey
- ¼ teaspoon garlic powder

Instructions

In a shallow dish, drizzle chicken with half of the olive oil, half of the lemon juice, salt, and pepper.

Heat a grill or grill pan over medium-high heat. Grill chicken 5 minutes on each side, or until no longer pink, or reaches an internal temperature of 165°F. Once chicken is cooked, remove from grill and slice into strips. Set aside.

In a large shallow serving dish, add spinach, strawberries, avocado, red onion, almonds, and mint. Top with chicken and feta.

In a small bowl, whisk together remaining lemon juice, remaining olive oil, honey, and garlic powder. Drizzle over salad and serve immediately.

380 calories • 15 g carbohydrate • 5 g fiber • 22 g fat (3 g saturated fat) • 32 g protein • 400 mg sodium

Kale and Edamame Power Salad with Maple Almond Dressing

This salad is loaded with antioxidant-rich vegetables. Almonds, avocado, and olive oil provide a good source of heart healthy fats.

Serves 4

Ingredients

Maple Almond Dressing

⅓ cup maple almond butter

⅓ cup apple cider vinegar

2 tablespoons water

1 teaspoon extra virgin olive oil

2 teaspoons maple syrup

¼ teaspoon ground ginger

½ teaspoon garlic powder

¼ teaspoon kosher salt

¼ teaspoon freshly ground black pepper

Instructions

Place all ingredients in a food processor. Process 1 minute or until smooth.

¼ cup serving:

110 calories • 7 g carbohydrate • 2 g fiber • 9 g fat (1 g saturated fat) • 3 g protein • 150 mg sodium

Ingredients

Kale and Edamame Power Salad

8 cups kale, chopped

2 teaspoons extra virgin olive oil

1 cup frozen edamame, thawed

1 cup shredded carrots

½ red bell pepper, chopped

¼ small red onion, cut into thin slices (about ¼ cup)

1 avocado, diced

1 cup zucchini, cut into 1 inch pieces

3 tablespoons slivered almonds

¼ cup dried cranberries

1 cup maple almond dressing

Instructions

Place kale in a large bowl. Drizzle with olive oil and rub with your hands.

Add edamame, carrots, bell pepper, red onion, avocado, zucchini, almonds, and cranberries. Drizzle salad with maple almond dressing.

Toss well and serve.

330 calories • 33 g carbohydrate • 11 g fiber • 20 g fat (2 g saturated fat) • 13 g protein • 270 mg sodium

Vegetarian Taco Salad with Creamy Cilantro Lime Dressing

This filling salad is full of veggies, fiber, and protein. The Greek yogurt dressing is so creamy, you won't miss the sour cream.

Serves 2

Ingredients

Vegetarian Taco Salad:
- **4** cups mixed field greens
- **1** teaspoon canola oil
- **2** tablespoons red onion, diced
- **½** jalapeño pepper, seeded and diced
- **1** cup canned unsalted pinto beans, rinsed and drained
- **½** teaspoon Mexican chili powder
- **½** teaspoon cumin
- **¼** teaspoon garlic powder
- **½** red or orange bell pepper, sliced into matchsticks
- **½** cup grape tomatoes, halved
- **½** avocado, sliced
- **2** tablespoons picante style salsa
- **¼** cup cheddar cheese, shredded
- **1** scallion (green parts only), sliced
- **12** whole grain, unsalted tortilla chips
- **½** lime, sliced in wedges

Instructions

Divide greens between two dinner plates and set aside.

In a small frying pan, heat oil over medium heat. Add onions and jalapeño and cook until softened, about 3 minutes. Stir in beans, chili powder, cumin, and garlic powder. Cook 3 minutes or until beans are warm.

Add beans evenly into the center of the greens on each plate. Top each with bell pepper, tomatoes, avocado, salsa, and cheese.

Drizzle dressing evenly over salads. Top with scallions. Serve with tortilla chips and lime wedges.

Ingredients

Instructions

Cilantro Lime Dressing:
2 tablespoons Greek yogurt
1 teaspoon extra virgin olive oil
Juice of **1** lime
1 tablespoon cilantro,
    finely chopped
1/8 teaspoon kosher salt
1/8 teaspoon freshly ground
    black pepper

To make dressing, in a small
bowl, whisk together yogurt, olive
oil, lime juice, cilantro, salt, and
pepper.

390 calories • 46 g carbohydrate • 15 g fiber • 16 g fat (4 g saturated fat) • 20 g protein • 440 mg sodium

Asian Cobb Salad

This favorite American salad gets a healthy makeover.
We've swapped the bacon and bleu cheese for oranges
and almonds to make this a PCOS friendly dish.

Makes 4 servings

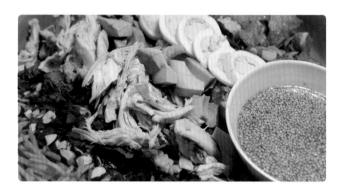

Ingredients

Sesame Dressing:
¼ cup rice wine vinegar
1 teaspoon fresh ginger, minced
1 teaspoon liquid amino acids
1 tablespoon creamy
   peanut butter
1 tablespoon canola oil
2 teaspoons sesame oil
1 teaspoon honey
¼ teaspoon garlic powder
2 teaspoons sesame seeds

Instructions

Place all ingredients in a small
mixing bowl and whisk well.

3 tablespoons:
60 calories • 2 g carbohydrate • < 1 g fiber, 6 g fat (< 1 g saturated fat) • <1 g protein • 75 mg sodium

Ingredients

Asian Cobb Salad:

8 cups romaine lettuce, chopped
2 ¼ cups rotisserie chicken, pulled from bone, skin removed (about ½ chicken)
1 ½ cup shredded carrots
2 cara cara or navel oranges, peeled
3 tablespoons unsalted slivered almonds
1 avocado, diced
2 hard-boiled eggs, sliced
¼ cup fresh cilantro, roughly chopped
2 green onions, diced

For sesame dressing, please see previous page.

Instructions

Place romaine lettuce in the bottom of a large, shallow bowl or serving dish. Add remaining ingredients over top and toss with sesame dressing.

Serve immediately.

390 calories • 23 g carbohydrate • 8 g fiber • 20 g fat (3 g saturated fat) • 35 g protein • 450 mg sodium

Kale Caesar Salad with Shrimp and Chickpea Croutons

The traditional Caesar salad is made with Romaine lettuce and creamy dressing. We give it a healthy makeover by substituting kale and a Greek yogurt based dressing for a delicious meal.

Serves 4

Ingredients

Caesar Dressing:

1 cup Greek yogurt
1 clove of garlic, chopped
Juice of **1** lemon
½ teaspoon mustard
1 tablespoon extra virgin olive oil
½ teaspoon freshly ground
    black pepper
1 teaspoon anchovy paste
3 tablespoons parmesan cheese
1 tablespoon water

Instructions

Place all ingredients in a food processor. Process 1 minute or until smooth.

2 tablespoons:
50 calories • 2 g carbohydrate • < 1 g fiber • 3.5 g fat (< .5 g saturated fat) • 4 g protein • 240 mg sodium

Ingredients

Kale Caesar Salad:

1, (14 ounce) can garbanzo
   beans, rinsed and drained
2 tablespoons extra virgin
   olive oil, divided
¼ teaspoon kosher salt, divided
½ teaspoon freshly ground black
   pepper, divided
8 cups kale, chopped
1 pound shrimp, peeled
   and divined
3 tablespoons shredded
   parmesan cheese
Caesar salad dressing

Instructions

Preheat oven to 375°F.

To make croutons, spread
garbanzo beans out on a large
baking sheet. Toss with ½ of olive
oil, half of salt and pepper. Bake
in oven for 15 to 20 minutes or
until beans start to brown.
Remove from oven.

Heat grill or grill pan on high
heat.

Drizzle shrimp with remaining
olive oil. Season with remaining
salt and black pepper to taste.
Grill shrimp for 2 to 3 minutes on
each side or until shrimp turn
pink.

In a large, shallow bowl combine
kale, shrimp, chickpea croutons,
and cheese.

Drizzle with Caesar dressing.
Toss well to combine.

350 calories • 28 g carbohydrate • 9 g fiber • 15.5 g fat (2.5 g saturated fat) • 30 g protein • 580 mg sodium

Tropical Tuna Chopped Salad

A healthier version of the classic tuna salad prepared with mayonnaise, this recipe incorporates heart healthy fats from olive oil and avocado.

Serves 2

Ingredients

- **1**, (5 ounce) can wild albacore tuna
- **1** cup mango, diced
- **½** red bell pepper, diced
- **¼** avocado, diced
- **1** large carrot, cut into match sticks
- **½** jalapeño, seeded and finely diced
- **2** tablespoons cilantro, roughly chopped
- **1** green onion, chopped
- **2** tablespoons extra virgin olive oil
- Zest and juice of **1** lime
- **¼** teaspoon kosher salt
- **½** teaspoon freshly ground black pepper
- **1** head romaine lettuce, chopped

Instructions

In a medium mixing bowl, combine tuna, mango, red pepper, avocado, carrot, jalapeño, cilantro, green onion, oil, lemon zest and juice, salt, and pepper. Mix well.

Divide chopped romaine lettuce among two plates. Top with chopped tuna salad. Serve immediately.

Tips

▸ Use pre-cut carrots to save time.
▸ To use as leftovers, store lettuce and tuna salad separately.

360 calories • 28 g carbohydrate • 11 g fiber • 18 g fat (2.5 g saturated fat) • 27 g protein • 390 mg sodium

Wheat Berry Antipasti Salad

Wheat berries are the whole grain form of wheat that haven't undergone any processing. They're full of fiber, folic acid, protein, and vitamins and provide a chewy, nutty flavor.

Serves 3

Ingredients

2 cups wheat berries, cooked

1 cup grape tomatoes, halved

2 roasted red peppers, diced (about two tablespoons)

¾ cup mini fresh mozzarella balls (bocconcini)

1, (6 ounce) jar marinated artichoke hearts, drained and roughly chopped

2 tablespoons fresh basil, roughly chopped

2 tablespoons extra virgin olive oil

⅛ teaspoon kosher salt

¼ teaspoon freshly ground black pepper

2 tablespoons balsamic vinegar

1 teaspoon honey

6 cups arugula

Instructions

Combine, wheat berries, grape tomatoes, peppers, mozzarella, artichokes, olive oil, salt, and pepper. Mix well.

In a small bowl, whisk together balsamic vinegar and honey. Set aside.

Top 3 plates with 2 cups of arugula. Evenly distribute wheat berry salad on top of greens. Drizzle each salad with balsamic mixture.

Tips

▸ Wheat berries can be made ahead of time. Just cover and refrigerate for up to 2 days or freeze for up to 1 month.

▸ For leftovers, pack arugula separately to avoid wilting and combine when you're ready to eat.

370 calories • 36 g carbohydrate • 5 g fiber • 19 g fat (5 g saturated fat) • 16 g protein • 370 mg sodium

Salade Niçoise

This classic French salad is a perfect meal. It has a balance of healthy fats, fiber, carbohydrates, and antioxidants.

Serves 3

Ingredients

Dressing:
Juice of **1** lemon
Zest of **1** lemon
2 tablespoons extra virgin olive oil
1 tablespoon Dijon Mustard
¼ teaspoon freshly ground black pepper

Instructions

To make dressing, in a small mixing bowl, whisk together lemon juice, zest, oil, mustard, and black pepper. Drizzle over top of salad. Mix well.

Serve immediately.

Ingredients

Salade Nicoise:

½ pound fingerling potatoes, boiled until tender

1 tablespoon red wine vinegar

1 tablespoon shallots, diced

1 tablespoon fresh parsley, roughly chopped

8 ounces hericot verts (French-style green beans), boiled until tender and cut in half

4 cups mixed baby greens

1 cup cherry tomatoes, halved

½ cup Nicoise or Kalamata olives

½ cup radishes, sliced

2 hard boiled eggs, thinly sliced

2, (4 ounce) cans tuna fish, drained

¼ cup chopped basil leaves

¼ cup scallions, diced

Instructions

Slice cooked potatoes into 2-inch pieces. In a medium bowl, toss potatoes with red wine vinegar, shallots,and parsley. Set aside.

Place mixed baby greens in a large, shallow serving bowl. Add potatoes, beans, tomatoes, olives, radishes, eggs, and tuna. Garnish with basil leaves and scallions.

Tips

▸ If you like anchovies, they are a great addition to this classic.
▸ Look for low sodium or no salt added tuna fish.

300 calories • 22 g carbohydrate • 5 g fiber • 14 g fat (2.5 g saturated fat) • 22 g protein • 357 mg sodium

Nonno's Tomato Salad

A summer favorite in our Italian household,
this salad is a classic Mediterranean side dish.

Serves 4

Ingredients

2 cups thinly sliced tomatoes
(about 2 medium beefsteak
tomatoes)
⅛ teaspoon kosher salt
¼ cup chopped red onion
½ cup chopped green pepper
¼ cup good extra virgin olive oil
2 tablespoons red wine vinegar

Instructions

Place tomatoes in a medium
sized bowl. Sprinkle with salt.
Let sit for 5 minutes. Add onion,
green pepper, olive oil, and
vinegar. Mix well.

Tip

▸ Add some fresh mozzarella to make this salad a light meal.

140 calories • 4 g carbohydrate • 2 g fiber • 14 g fat (2 g saturated fat) • 1 g protein • 92 mg sodium

Butter Lettuce Salad with Apple Cider Vinaigrette

Butter lettuce is so delicate, it pairs best with a light dressing. Apple cider vinegar is linked to improving insulin resistance and blood sugar levels.

Serves 4

Ingredients

Apple Cider Vinaigrette
Makes ½ cup
- **1** tablespoon balsamic vinegar
- **1** tablespoon apple cider vinegar
- **2** teaspoons honey
- ¼ cup peanut oil

Instructions

In a small bowl, whisk together all ingredients.

2 tablespoons:

131 calories • 3 g carbohydrate • < 1 g fiber • 14 g fat (2 g saturated fat) •< 1 g protein • 116 mg sodium

Ingredients

Butter Lettuce Salad
- **4** cups butter lettuce
- **1** medium Granny Smith apple, thinly sliced
- ⅓ cup chopped walnut halves
- ½ cup Apple Cider Vinaigrette

Instructions

Place lettuce in a medium bowl.
Top with apples and walnuts.
Add dressing and mix well.

Serve immediately.

Tip

 Instead of whisking, place ingredients in a closed bottle or jar and shake well to combine.

214 calories, 10 g carbohydrate, 2 g fiber, 19 g fat (3 g saturated fat), 1 g protein, 117 mg sodium

Spinach Salad with Cinnamon Orange Vinaigrette

This green salad boasts strong flavors of cinnamon and orange. Hemp hearts give a rich nutty flavor with tender crunch and along with sunflower oil, provides a good dose of heart healthy fats.

Serves 6

Ingredients

Cinnamon Orange Vinaigrette:

¼ cup sunflower oil
¼ cup rice wine vinegar
1 ½ teaspoons ground cinnamon
½ cup freshly squeezed orange juice
2 teaspoons orange zest

Instructions

Combine all ingredients in a small bowl. Whisk well to combine.

Tip

▸ Instead of whisking, shake dressing well in a closed bottle or jar to combine.

2 tablespoons:

71 calories • 2 g carbohydrate • < 1 g fiber • 7 g fat (1 g saturated fat) • < 1 g protein • < 1 mg sodium

Ingredients

Spinach Salad
6 cups baby spinach leaves
4 tablespoons hemp hearts
½ large orange, peeled and cut
    into 1 inch slices
½ cup cinnamon orange
    vinaigrette dressing

Instructions

Place spinach leaves in a serving
bowl. Top with hemp hearts and
oranges. Add dressing. Mix well.

Serve immediately.

Tip
 Look for hemp hearts in the nuts and seeds section of your
grocery store.

206 calories • 8 g carbohydrate • 3 g fiber • 18 g fat (2 g saturated fat) • 4 g protein • 24 mg sodium

Tuscan Arugula Salad

This simple salad is an easy way to add more
vegetables and omega-3 fats to your meal.

Serves 4

Ingredients

4 cups arugula
⅓ cup walnut halves
2 Roma tomatoes, sliced
8 pitted olives
2 tablespoons balsamic vinegar
1 teaspoon freshly ground
  black pepper
2 tablespoons freshly grated
  parmesan cheese

Instructions

Place arugula in a serving bowl.
Top with walnuts, tomatoes, and
olives. Add balsamic vinegar and
pepper. Mix well. Top with cheese
and serve immediately.

118 calories, 6 g carbohydrate, 2 g fiber, 10 g fat (1 g saturated fat), 3 g protein, 313 mg sodium

Field Greens Salad with Lemon Dijon Vinaigrette

This simple salad is a great way to add a serving of green vegetables to any meal.

Serves 4

Ingredients

- **5** cups mixed baby field greens
- **2** tablespoons extra virgin olive oil
- **1** tablespoon white wine vinegar
- Juice of ½ a lemon
- **1** tablespoon Dijon mustard
- **1** teaspoon honey
- ¼ teaspoon freshly ground black pepper
- ¼ teaspoon kosher salt

Instructions

Place mixed greens in a large bowl.

In a small mixing bowl, whisk together remaining ingredients. Drizzle vinaigrette over salad and toss well to coat leaves.

Tip

► Increase the nutrient content of this salad by adding your favorite vegetables, nuts or seeds.

80 calories • 4 g carbohydrate • 2 g fiber • 7 g fat (1 g saturated fat) • < 1 g protein • 150 mg sodium

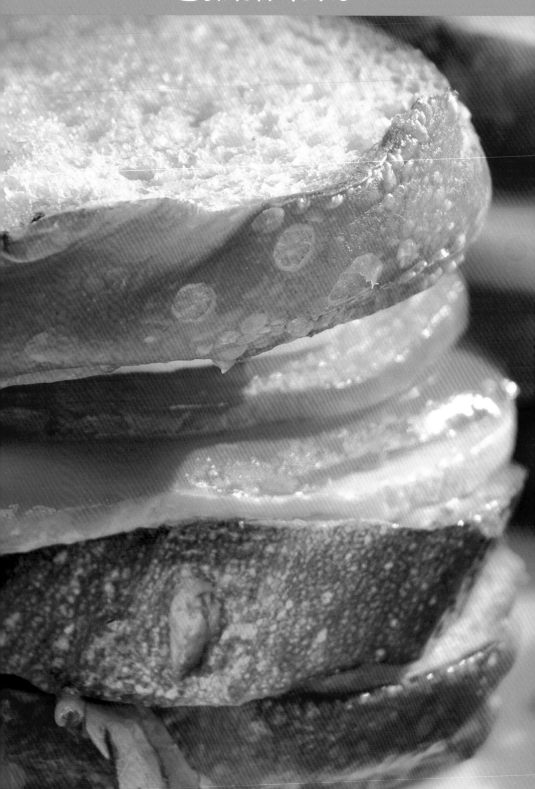

Sandwiches

Five-Layer Turkey Sandwich with Cannellini Bean Spread

This turkey sandwich version is loaded with fiber, protein, and flavor.

Makes 1 sandwich

Ingredients

1 whole wheat pocket-less pita
3 tablespoons cannellini bean, lemon and herb spread **(see next recipe)**
8 cucumber slices
3 ounces turkey breast
¼ cup arugula
2 tomato slices

Instructions

Cut pita in half, making two half-moons.

Spread cannellini bean spread evenly on both halves. Layer cucumber, turkey, arugula, and tomato on one pita half. Place other pita on top and serve immediately.

350 calories • 40 g carbohydrate • 7 g fiber • 7 g fat (1 g saturated fat) • 34 g protein • 403 mg sodium

Cannellini Bean, Lemon and Herb Spread

This delicious healthy spread is full of fiber and flavor.

Makes 8 servings

Ingredients

1, (15 ounce) can cannellini
  beans, rinsed and drained
2 tablespoons fresh basil,
  roughly chopped
1 tablespoon fresh Italian flat
  leaf parsley, roughly chopped
2 tablespoons extra virgin
  olive oil
2 teaspoons lemon zest
1 tablespoon fresh lemon juice
¼ teaspoon kosher salt
Freshly ground black pepper
  to taste

Instructions

Combine ingredients in a food processor.

Process 30 seconds or until smooth.

Refrigerate in an airtight container for up to 1 week.

Tip
▸ Can be served as a dip with fresh veggies.

3 tablespoons:
90 calories • 11 g carbohydrate • 3 g fiber • 4 g fat (<1 g saturated fat) • 4 g protein • 75 mg sodium

Egg Salad Sandwich

This egg salad uses a fraction of the mayo a traditional recipe calls for. We've cut the saturated fat while leaving flavor and protein.

Serves 2

Ingredients

3 eggs, hard boiled and diced
1 tablespoon olive oil mayonnaise
1 tablespoon whole grain mustard
½ teaspoon spicy yellow mustard
½ teaspoon chives, diced
¼ teaspoon kosher salt
¼ teaspoon freshly ground black pepper
4 slices low sodium, sprouted grain bread
4 romaine lettuce leaves

Instructions

In a medium mixing bowl, combine eggs, mayo, mustards, chives, salt, and pepper. Mix well.

Divide salad among two slices of bread. Top with lettuce leaves and remaining slices of bread.

Serve immediately.

Tip

▸ When boiling eggs, add extras to the pot to save for later in the week.

310 calories • 32 g carbohydrate • 7 g fiber • 12 g fat (3 g saturated fat) • 18 g protein • 490 mg sodium

Mayo-Less
Chicken Salad Sandwich

A healthier version of a lunch classic, we've substituted
Greek yogurt for traditional mayonnaise. Not only is this
sandwich lower in saturated fat, but it's higher in protein.

Serves 2

Ingredients

- 1 ½ cups pulled rotisserie chicken, chopped
- 1 tablespoon plain Greek yogurt
- 1 tablespoon Dijon mustard
- 1 tablespoon celery, finely chopped
- 1 scallion, green and white parts, diced
- 1 teaspoon parsley, roughly chopped
- ⅛ teaspoon kosher salt
- ¼ teaspoon freshly ground black pepper
- 4 slices sprouted grain bread
- 4 Romaine lettuce leaves

Instructions

In a medium mixing bowl, combine chicken, yogurt, mustard, celery, scallions, parsley, salt, and pepper. Mix well.

Divide salad among two slices of bread. Top with lettuce leaves and remaining slices of bread.

Serve immediately.

Tip

 ► For variety, add fresh herbs like cilantro or basil for different flavors.

380 calories • 33 g carbohydrate • 7 g fiber • 6 g fat (1 g saturated fat) • 49 g protein • 530 mg sodium

Italian-Style Tuna Salad Wrap

Say goodbye to your typical tuna salad! Here's a much
healthier twist on a sandwich classic that leaves
out the mayo and packs a lot of flavor.

Serves 2

Ingredients

- 1, (5 ounce) can solid white tuna, drained
- 1 tablespoon Kalamata olives, finely diced
- ½ sweet red bell pepper, finely diced
- 1 tablespoon green onion, diced
- 2 sundried tomatoes, diced
- 1 teaspoon fresh parsley, roughly chopped
- ½ teaspoon freshly ground black pepper
- Juice from ½ a lemon
- 2 tablespoons extra virgin olive oil
- ½ cup arugula
- 2 whole wheat sandwich wraps

Instructions

In a medium mixing bowl, combine tuna, olives, pepper, onion, tomatoes, parsley, ground pepper, lemon juice and olive oil. Mix well.

Divide arugula between the two sandwich wraps. Place leaves in the center of the wrap and top each with half of the tuna mixture. Roll into a sandwich wrap and serve.

Tip

▸ This salad is also very tasty on top of mixed greens

380 calories • 33 g carbohydrate • 5 g fiber • 16 g fat (2.5 g saturated fat) • 27 g protein • 350 mg sodium

Edamame
Veggie Burgers

Mushrooms, walnuts, and edamame make
this burger so hearty, you won't miss the meat.

Serves 4

Ingredients

- **1** tablespoon plus **1** teaspoon canola oil
- **2** cups shiitake mushrooms, sliced
- **1** cup frozen shelled edamame, unthawed
- **1** clove garlic, roughly chopped
- ¾ cup shelled & peeled walnuts
- **1** tablespoon fresh parsley, roughly chopped
- **1** egg
- **1** teaspoon low sodium tamari or soy sauce
- ⅛ teaspoon ground ginger
- ⅛ teaspoon cumin
- ¼ cup whole wheat panko bread crumbs
- ½ teaspoon freshly ground black pepper

Instructions

Heat 1 teaspoon of oil in a small fry pan over medium-high heat. Add mushrooms. Sauté until mushrooms are just softened, 3 to 5 minutes.

In a food processor, combine mushrooms, edamame, garlic, walnuts, parsley, egg, tamari, ginger, cumin, panko and pepper. Process 30 minutes or until edamame and walnuts are finely chopped (don't over process or you may get a paste).

Form burgers into 4 patties. Heat remaining oil in a large skillet heat over medium heat. Add burgers. Cook until golden brown on each side, turning once, about 5 to 7 minutes.

Serve immediately.

Tips

▸ To save some prep time, look for sliced shiitake mushrooms in your supermarket.
▸ Serve these burgers over Romaine lettuce leaves or over a salad.

300 calories • 21 g carbohydrate • 6 g fiber • 20 g fat (2 g saturated fat) • 12 g protein • 260 mg sodium

Mediterranean Chicken Wrap

This heart healthy sandwich is sure to leave you satisfied. It's also a great way to sneak in a few servings of veggies for the day!

Serves 1

Ingredients

- **1** large whole wheat tortilla or sandwich wrap
- **1** tablespoon hummus
- **4** thinly sliced cucumber slices
- **¼** cup mixed greens
- **4** grape tomatoes, halved
- **1** tablespoon feta cheese
- **1** teaspoon diced red onion
- **4** ounces grilled chicken breast, diced
- **3** Kalamata olives, pitted and diced

Instructions

Spread hummus evenly over one side of wrap. Lay cucumber slices on top. Layer greens, tomatoes, cheese, onion, chicken and olives on top, keeping them towards the center.

Fold two sides halfway up wrap and begin to tightly roll beginning on either of the remaining sides.

Tip

▸ The grilled chicken prepared in the Grilled Chicken and Strawberry Spinach Salad works really well in this wrap.

300 calories • 30 g carbohydrate • 5 g fiber • 8 g fat (3 g saturated fat) • 27 g protein • 520 mg sodium

Vegetarian Reuben Sandwich

This traditional sandwich gets a healthy vegetarian makeover with seitan, mushrooms and caramelized onions. Seitan (pronounced "say-tan"), also called "wheat meat," is a high-protein, low fat food with a meaty texture and flavor. Look for it refrigerated in the organic department of your grocery store.

Makes 1 sandwich

Ingredients

- **2** teaspoons extra virgin olive oil, plus **1** teaspoon
- ½ cup chopped onion
- **1** sliced portabella mushroom
- **4** ounces seitan, drained and thinly sliced
- ½ teaspoon garlic powder
- ⅛ teaspoon kosher salt
- ⅛ teaspoon freshly ground pepper
- **1** tablespoon mayonnaise (olive-oil based one)
- **1** teaspoon ketchup
- **1** teaspoon finely chopped dill pickle
- **2** slices sprouted grain bread
- **2** tablespoons sauerkraut, drained
- **1** ounce Swiss cheese

Instructions

In a large skillet, add 2 teaspoons of olive oil and onions. Cook over medium heat until almost caramelized, about 10 minutes. Add portabella mushroom slices, seitan, garlic powder, salt, and pepper. Mix well. Cook for 4 to 6 minutes, until seitan and mushrooms are cooked and onions are caramelized.

To make dressing, whisk together mayonnaise, ketchup, and pickle in small bowl.

Heat grill pan over medium-high heat. Lightly brush each slice of bread with remaining olive oil on one side.

Pile the seitan, onions and mushrooms on the bread (greased side down). Drizzle sandwich with dressing. Top with sauerkraut followed by cheese. Top with another slice of bread (greased side up). Place on grill.

Cook until cheese is melted and bread is toasted, about 2 to 3 minutes on each side.

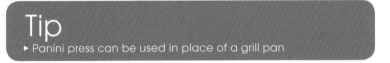

Tip

▸ Panini press can be used in place of a grill pan

448 calories • 26 g carbohydrate • 5 g fiber • 29 g fat (5 g saturated fat) • 23 g protein • 515 mg sodium

Spinach Turkey Burgers

A tastier and leaner alternative to traditional hamburgers, these turkey burgers are rich in iron and protein but low in fat.

Serves 4

Ingredients

- 1 pound ground turkey (93 to 95% lean)
- 1 garlic clove, minced
- ¾ cup frozen chopped spinach, thawed
- Zest of 1 lemon
- 1 egg
- ¼ teaspoon kosher salt
- ¼ teaspoon freshly ground black pepper
- 4 small whole wheat rolls
- 4 lettuce leaves (garnish)
- 4 tomato slices (garnish)
- 4 red onion slices (garnish)

Instructions

In a large bowl, combine turkey, garlic, spinach, lemon zest, egg, salt, and pepper. Mix well with hands. Form mixture into 4 patties.

Heat grill pan or grill to medium-high heat. Cook for 5 to 7 minutes on each side or until cooked throughout or reaches an internal temperature of 165°F.

Place cooked patties between rolls. Top with lettuce, tomato, onion and your favorite condiment.

Cook until cheese is melted and bread is toasted, about 2 to 3 minutes on each side.

Tip

▶ The Greek yogurt aioli from the Salmon Cakes recipe is a perfect condiment with this.

200 calories, 2 g carbohydrate, <1 g fiber, 11 g fat (3 g saturated fat), 24 g protein, 350 mg sodium

Ultimate Vegetable Sandwich

Bring on the veggies! This sandwich is loaded with grilled vegetables.
Sourdough is a fermented bread that has a lower glycemic index value
than most breads. Walnut pesto makes a yummy spread.

Serves 2

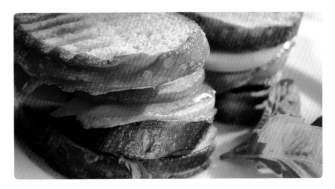

Ingredients

2 tablespoons extra virgin
olive oil, divided
1 small zucchini sliced on an
angle in half-inch thick slices
1 small yellow squash, sliced
on an angle in half-inch
thick slices
4 lengthwise strips of red pepper
4 slices red onion
¼ teaspoon kosher salt
½ teaspoon freshly ground
black pepper
4 slices sourdough bread
½ cup arugula
6 ounces fresh water-packed
mozzarella cheese,
drained, sliced
1 tablespoon Walnut Pesto

Instructions

Heat a grill pan over medium-high heat. Using a pastry
brush, brush half of oil on both
sides of the zucchini, squash,
red pepper, and onion slices.
Season with salt and pepper.
Place vegetables on a hot grill
and cook until they are tender.
Cool completely.

Once vegetables are done,
brush bread slices with olive oil
and grill on both sides. Spread
pesto on one side of bread slices.

To assemble sandwiches, start
with the bottom 2 slices of bread
(pesto side up). On each, place
arugula, stack 2 slices of zucchini, 2 slices of squash, 2 slices of
red pepper, and onion. Top with
mozzarella. Place remaining 2
bread slices (pesto side down)
on top.

625 calories • 45 g carbohydrate • 7 g fiber • 36 g fat (13 g saturated fat) • 36 g protein • 561 mg sodium

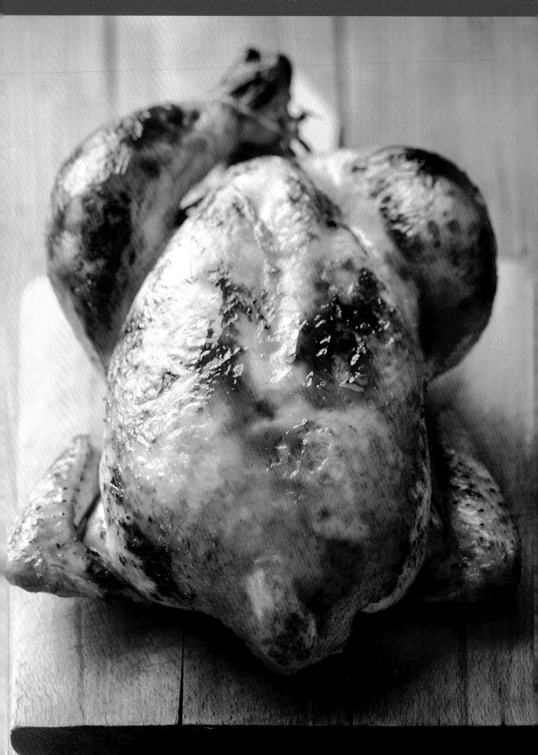

Sweet and Savory Roast Chicken

This flavorful roast chicken combines the sweet flavor of red grapes with the savory flavors of garlic, rosemary, and thyme.

Serves 5

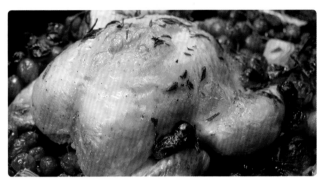

Ingredients

- **1** whole chicken, about 3 pounds (bone included)
- **1** tablespoon plus **1** teaspoon extra virgin olive oil, divided
- **½** teaspoon kosher salt, divided
- **½** teaspoon freshly ground black pepper
- **1** pound red seedless grapes, separated with stems in small bunches
- **2** red onions, cut in 2 inch wedges
- **1** tablespoon fresh rosemary, roughly chopped
- **1** tablespoon fresh thyme leaves, plus **6** to **8** full thyme sprigs
- **6** cloves of garlic, peeled

Instructions

Preheat oven to 400°F.

Rub chicken with half of the olive oil, half of the salt and half pepper. Place chicken in the center of a roasting pan.

In a medium bowl, toss grapes with remaining olive oil and salt, onion, rosemary, and thyme leaves.

Pour grape mixture around chicken in roasting pan. Add thyme sprigs and garlic in the cavity of the chicken. Roast 50 to 60 minutes or until meat thermometer reads 165°F at the thickest part of the chicken.

Remove chicken from oven and allow it to sit for 10 minutes before serving.

Tips

▸ Roasting times may vary depending on chicken size.
▸ Removing the skin before you eat it will reduce the total and saturated fat content.

420 calories • 18 g carbohydrate • 2 g fiber • 22 g fat (6 g saturated fat) • 37 g protein • 470 mg sodium

Sesame Ginger Glazed Salmon

Fatty fish like salmon are rich in omega-3 fatty acids, fats that are good for the brain and heart. They're also important for lowering inflammation. Ginger improves inflammation as well as digestion.

Serves 2, 6 ounce fillets

Ingredients

1 tablespoon toasted sesame oil plus **1** teaspoon
2 tablespoons rice wine vinegar
1 tablespoon low sodium soy sauce
¼ cup freshly squeezed orange juice
1 tablespoon freshly grated ginger
2 (6 ounce) boneless, skinless salmon fillets
1 tablespoon toasted sesame seeds

Instructions

Preheat oven to 400°F.

Combine 1 tablespoon sesame oil, vinegar, soy sauce, juice, and ginger in a shallow baking dish; whisk to blend. Add the salmon to the dish. Cover and let marinate at room temperature for 30 minutes, turning once half-way through the marinating time.

Heat an additional teaspoon of oil in an oven-safe nonstick skillet. Add fish to skillet (discard marinade) and cook 3 to 4 minutes over medium heat until lightly browned. Turn fish over and sprinkle with sesame seeds. Place skillet in oven and bake for 6 to 8 minutes or until fish is opaque throughout or reaches an internal temperature of 145°F.

Tips

▸ Wild caught salmon generally has less toxins than farm raised.
▸ Look for toasted sesame seeds at your local grocery store.

360 calories • 5 g carbohydrate • 1 g fiber • 21 g fat (3 g saturated fat) • 35 g protein • 292 mg sodium

Marinated Flank Steak

Flank steak is versatile, easy to prepare, and one of the leaner cuts of beef. This savory marinade makes for a sizzling and tasty meal. Thanks to culinary wizard and Registered Dietitian Moira Gledhill for sharing this delicious recipe.

Serves 6 (serving size: 4 ounces)

Ingredients

- **1** (1 ½ pounds) flank steak, trimmed
- **¼** cup chopped fresh rosemary (or 1 tablespoon dried rosemary, crushed)
- **1** tablespoon chopped fresh marjoram (or **1** teaspoon dried marjoram, crushed)
- **1** tablespoon chopped fresh oregano (or **1** teaspoon dried oregano, crushed)
- **1 ½** teaspoon smoked paprika
- **3** cloves minced garlic
- **1** teaspoon kosher salt
- **1** teaspoon crushed red pepper
- **1** teaspoon freshly ground black pepper
- **3** tablespoons extra virgin olive oil

Instructions

Preheat oven to 400°F.

Prepare steak by scoring both sides of the steak in a diamond pattern, making shallow cuts at 1 inch intervals, set aside.

In a small bowl, mix together rosemary, marjoram, oregano, paprika, garlic, salt, red and black pepper. Stir in oil until combined.

Place steak in a wide flat dish. Pour the marinade onto the steak. Cover and refrigerate for 8 hours (or up to 24 hours in advance).

Preheat grill to medium. Place steak directly on the grill (discard marinade) and cook for 17 to 19 minutes, or to preferred doneness, turning once.

Remove steak from grill. Cover and let stand for 10 minutes. To serve, slice steak thinly across the grain.

Tip
▸ This marinade is suitable and delicious with any type of grilled red meat.

360 calories • < 1 g carbohydrate • < 1 g fiber, 25 g fat (9 g saturated fat) • 31 g protein • 157 mg sodium

Lemon Thyme
Baked Chicken Breasts

This moist and delicious dish adds protein
and heart healthy fats to your dinner plate.

Serves 4

Ingredients

1 ½ pounds skinless
   chicken breasts
1 tablespoon fresh lemon juice
¼ teaspoon kosher salt
3 tablespoons extra virgin
   olive oil, divided
6 cloves of garlic, cut in quarters
6 - 8 fresh thyme sprigs
½ lemon, sliced
¼ teaspoon freshly ground
   black pepper

Instructions

Preheat oven to 350°F.

Place chicken breasts in a quart
sized zip lock bag. Pound chicken
with a meat tenderizer until ½
inch thick.

Add lemon juice, salt, and
½ of the olive oil into bag and
seal well. Massage bag to coat
chicken.

Remove chicken from bag and
place in oven safe casserole dish.
Add garlic. Place thyme sprigs on
chicken and cover with lemon
slices. Drizzle remaining olive oil
over chicken. Season generously
with freshly ground pepper.

Bake 30 minutes or until chicken
reaches an internal temperature
of 165°F.

Tip
▸ To create a PCOS friendly dinner, pair this chicken with a
   simple arugula salad and barley risotto.

300 calories, 2 g carbohydrate, 0 g fiber, 15 g fat (2.5 g saturated fat), 39 g protein, 80 mg sodium

Savory Roast Turkey Breast

Turkey doesn't have to be reserved for Thanksgiving.
Enjoy this lean, high protein food all year round
on its own, in sandwiches or salads.

Serves 4

Ingredients

4 pounds half turkey breast, bone in and skin on
1 ½ teaspoon fresh rosemary
1 teaspoon thyme
1 teaspoon sage, chopped
½ teaspoon kosher salt, divided
1 teaspoon freshly ground black pepper, plus **½** teaspoon
2 teaspoons lemon zest
2 tablespoons unsalted butter, softened
1 teaspoon extra virgin olive oil

Instructions

Preheat oven to 325°F.

Pat dry turkey using paper towels.

In a small bowl, combine rosemary, thyme, sage, half of salt, 1 teaspoon pepper, zest, butter, and oil to form a paste. Reserve 1 tablespoon of paste. Rub paste under the skin as far as possible. Rub outside of skin with remaining paste. Season with remaining salt and pepper.

Place on rack in roasting pan. Cover with foil, making a tent (sides should be open). Cook 60 to 90 minutes or until reaches an internal temperature of 165°F.

Let rest for 10 to 15 minutes. Slice and serve.

Tip
▸ Save leftover turkey to use in our Five-Layer Turkey Sandwich recipe.

253 calories • 0 g carbohydrate • 0 g fiber • 13 g fat (5 g saturated fat) • 32 g protein • 650 mg sodium

Shrimp Tacos

This meal makes a great dish for entertaining guests or a quiet dinner at home.

Serves 4 (makes 12 tacos)

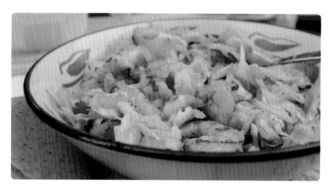

Ingredients

1 pound large shrimp, peeled and deveined

¼ cup extra virgin olive oil plus **1** tablespoon

1 teaspoon ground chili powder

1 tablespoon ground cumin

½ teaspoon kosher salt

3 slices of pineapple (½ inch thick, length of pineapple)

3 cups shredded cabbage

½ cup grated carrots

1 avocado, diced

¼ cup freshly chopped cilantro

⅓ cup fresh lime juice (about **2** limes)

12 corn tortillas

Instructions

Preheat grill.

Thread shrimp on skewers. In a small bowl whisk 1 tablespoon of olive oil, chili powder, cumin, and salt. Brush onto both sides of shrimp. Grill shrimp over low heat until golden brown and slightly charred, about 2 to 3 minutes per side.

Grill pineapple over low heat until golden brown, about 2 to 3 minutes per side. Dice pineapple and place in large bowl. Add cabbage, carrots, avocado, cilantro, remaining olive oil, and lime juice. Mix well. Starting from the bottom, slide shrimp off skewers into bowl. Toss to combine. Serve with warm corn tortillas.

Tips

▸ Use pre-shredded cabbage and carrots to save time.
▸ A large non-stick skillet can also be used to cook shrimp.
▸ Place tortillas on grill for 1 to 2 minutes to warm.

600 calories • 53 g carbohydrate • 10 g fiber • 29 g fat (4 g saturated fat) • 33 g protein • 329 mg sodium

Slow-Cooker
Stuffed Peppers

Most stuffed peppers are full of rice making them
high in carbohydrates. These peppers cut the carbs
in half and are ready for you when you get home!

Serves 5

Ingredients

5 bell peppers
2 ½ cups cauliflower florets,
   (**1** cup riced cauliflower)
1 pound Italian-Style chicken
   sausage, removed from
   casing
½ cup marinara sauce
½ cup chopped walnuts
½ cup grated parmesan cheese
1 egg
¼ cup whole wheat panko
   bread crumbs
⅛ teaspoon kosher salt
¼ teaspoon freshly ground
   black pepper
1 cup water

Instructions

Remove core and seeds from
peppers. Reserve pepper tops
and set aside.

Pulse cauliflower florets in a
food processor until it resembles
rice. Measure out 1 cup of riced
cauliflower.

In a large bowl combine 1 cup
of riced cauliflower, chicken
sausage, marinara, walnuts,
cheese, egg, bread crumbs,
salt, and pepper. Use hands to
mix well.

Fill peppers with meat mixture.
Place filled peppers in the
bottom of a 6 quart slow-cooker
(peppers should fit tightly and
be able to stand up). Place
pepper tops over meat mixture.
Pour water in the bottom of the
slow-cooker.

Cook on low for 8 hours.

Tip
▸ Look for chicken sausage and marinara sauce varieties with
  less than 400mg of sodium.

300 calories • 18 g carbohydrate • 5 g fiber • 12 g fat (4.5 g saturated fat) • 20 g protein • 530 mg sodium

Halibut with Walnut Pesto

Halibut is a firm, white fish from the cold waters of the Atlantic and Pacific. Making this pesto with walnuts instead of traditional pine nuts, increases its omega-3 content. Preparing the pesto ahead of time and freezing it makes this meal quick, easy and delicious all year round.

Serves 2 fillets

Ingredients

2, 6 ounce skinless halibut fillets
1 tablespoon extra virgin olive oil
⅛ teaspoon kosher salt
⅛ teaspoon freshly
   ground pepper

Instructions

Preheat grill. Prepare the halibut by brushing on olive oil. Sprinkle with salt and pepper.

Grill the halibut over direct heat until browned on the first side, about 3 to 5 minutes. Turn fish and cook until browned on the second side, about 3 to 4 minutes. Fish should be opaque or reach an internal temperature of 140°F.

Top each fillet with 1 tablespoon of walnut pesto.
(see next recipe for pesto)

Tips
▸ Any fish can be substituted for halibut.
▸ To flip the fish without it falling apart or sticking to the grill, cook in a hinged grill basket.

340 calories • 1 g carbohydrate • < 1 g fiber • 20 g fat (3 g saturated fat) • 39 g protein • 358 mg sodium

Walnut Pesto

Makes 1 ½ cups

Ingredients

½ cup chopped walnuts
6 cloves garlic
3 cups fresh sweet basil, packed
½ teaspoon kosher salt
½ teaspoon freshly
   ground pepper
1 cup good quality extra
   virgin olive oil
½ cup freshly grated
   parmesan cheese

Instructions

To make pesto, place walnuts and garlic in a food processor. Pulse for 30 seconds. Scrape sides. Add basil, salt, and pepper. With the processor running, add oil and process until pesto is pureed. Scrape sides. Add parmesan cheese and puree for 30 seconds.

Tips

▸ Pesto can be used as a sandwich spread, mixed with pasta, tossed with vegetables or as a substitute for pizza sauce.
▸ Use this pesto for the Red Pepper and Pesto Egg Sandwich recipe.
▸ Freeze leftover pesto in ice cube trays and transfer to freezer bag. Simply thaw before use. One ice cube of pesto = 1 tablespoon.

1 tablespoon:
107 calories, 1 g carbohydrate, < 1 g fiber, 11 g fat (2 g saturated fat), 1 g protein, 57 mg sodium

Spicy Orange Sesame Chicken with Broccoli and Carrots

This chicken stir-fry with a kick recipe is shared by our friend Susan Adams, Registered Dietitian and Assistant Professor of Nutrition at LaSalle University.

Serves 4

Ingredients

2 teaspoons toasted
  sesame seeds
⅔ cup freshly squeezed
  orange juice
¼ cup water
½ teaspoon kosher salt
2 teaspoons balsamic vinegar
1 tablespoon cornstarch
3 tablespoons olive oil
2 cloves minced garlic
2 tablespoons minced shallot
Peeled zest of **1** large orange
  (no white pith)
¼ teaspoon red pepper flakes
1 pound skinless, boneless
  chicken breasts, cut
  in small cubes
1 large head of broccoli,
  separated into small florets
4 - 5 large carrots, sliced thin
  on the diagonal

Instructions

To toast sesame seeds, spread on a baking dish and bake in a 325°F oven until brown and fragrant (about 10-15 minutes).

Mix together the orange juice, water, salt, and balsamic vinegar until blended. Whisk in cornstarch until completely blended. Set aside.

Heat oil in a large frying pan or wok over medium heat. Sauté the garlic, shallots, orange zest, and red pepper flakes until the garlic and shallots have softened, stirring frequently. Add chicken and sauté until completely cooked and slightly brown or reaches an internal temperature of 165°F. Add the broccoli and carrots and sauté for 2 minutes, stirring frequently.

Add the orange juice mixture and stir until thickened. Cover pan and steam for 2 to 3 minutes or until the vegetables are crisp tender.

Sprinkle with sesame seeds and serve immediately.

Tips

▸ Serve over ½ cup brown rice if desired.
▸ Make sure vegetables are uniform size to cook evenly.
▸ To save time, look for toasted sesame seeds at your grocery store.

300 calories • 15 g carbohydrate • 3 g fiber • 14 g fat (2 g saturated fat) • 28 g protein • 410 mg sodium

Pecan-Crusted Trout

Trout is a mild flavored freshwater fish that is rich in omega-3 fats.

Serves 2

Ingredients

Cooking spray
¼ cup pecans
¼ cup unsweetened shredded
    coconut
½ teaspoon extra virgin olive oil
⅛ teaspoon kosher salt
⅛ teaspoon freshly
    ground pepper
2, 6 ounce trout fillets (skin intact)
Lemon wedges

Instructions

Preheat oven to 400°F.

Spray a baking pan with cooking spray. Place pecans in a food processor and grind until fine. Add coconut and mix well. Transfer to large plate.

Using a pastry brush, brush flesh side of fish with oil. Sprinkle fish with salt and pepper. Dip 1 fillet into almond mixture to coat with nuts, pressing down. Transfer to baking pan, pecan side up. Repeat with remaining fillet.

Bake for 10 to 12 minutes or until fish flakes easily. Serve with lemon wedges.

Tip
▸ Pineapple mango salsa works great as a topping.

378 calories • 7 g carbohydrate • 2 g fiber • 22 g fat (6 g saturated fat) • 38 g protein • 327 mg sodium

Spicy Cilantro Lime Chicken

Chili powder, jalapeno, garlic, and cumin give this chicken some serious heat! Thanks to Registered Dietitian and culinary wizard Moira Gledhill for sharing this favorite dish!

Serves 4

Ingredients

1 pound boneless, skinless chicken breasts
Juice from **2** limes, divided
5 garlic cloves
½ tablespoon cumin
1 teaspoon chili powder
¼ cup lite mayonnaise (olive oil based)
¼ cup non-fat Greek yogurt
1 jalapeño (seeds and stems removed)
1 cup freshly chopped cilantro
⅛ teaspoon kosher salt
⅛ teaspoon freshly ground black pepper

Instructions

Place the chicken in a large Ziploc bag. Add ½ of lime juice, 3 garlic cloves, cumin, and chili powder. With bag sealed, massage chicken with marinade and refrigerate for at least one hour (or up to 8 hours in advance).

Preheat grill to medium. Place chicken on grill (discard marinade) and cook until juices run clear or reaches an internal temperature of 165°F. Let the chicken rest for 10 minutes.

To make the sauce, in a small bowl blend the remaining lime juice, garlic, mayonnaise, yogurt, jalapeño, cilantro, salt, and pepper until smooth. Set aside.

Top chicken with one tablespoon of green cilantro sauce and serve.

Tip

▸ To prepare this recipe using a whole free range chicken, follow the steps above. Once grill is hot, place the cavity of a whole chicken onto an opened can of beer. The chicken and the beer should be able to stand on the grill without support. For best results grill the whole chicken using indirect heat until the juices run clear (up to at least 1 hour or internal temperature of 175°F). Serve sliced chicken alongside the cilantro sauce.

247 calories • 5 g carbohydrate • 1 g fiber • 10 g fat (2 g saturated fat) • 36 g protein • 188 mg sodium

Mediterranean Tuna Steaks

Tuna steaks are high in protein and rich in heart healthy omega-3 fats. This dish combines the delightful flavors of lemon, garlic, and basil.

Serves 3

Ingredients

2 tablespoons extra virgin olive oil, divided
3 tablespoons lemon juice
1 teaspoon lemon zest
1 clove of garlic, minced
⅓ cup Italian flat leaf parsley, finely chopped
⅓ cup fresh basil, finely chopped
⅛ teaspoon kosher salt, divided
¼ teaspoon freshly ground black pepper, divided
3 tuna steaks (4 ounces each)

Instructions

In a small bowl, combine 1 tablespoon olive oil, lemon juice and zest, garlic, parsley, basil, and half of salt and pepper. Whisk well and set aside.

Brush tuna steaks on both sides with 1 tablespoon of olive oil and season with remaining salt and pepper.

Heat a grill or grill pan on high heat. Add steaks. Cook 3 minutes on each side or until tuna reaches an internal temperature of 145°F.

Place steaks on plate and top with two tablespoons of lemon and herb mixture.

Serve immediately.

230 calories, 3 g carbohydrate, 0 g fiber, 13 g fat (2 g saturated fat), 26 g protein, 400 mg sodium

Pork with Apples and Carrots

This recipe is shared by our friend Susan Dopart, MS, RD, CDE from her book *A Recipe for Life by the Doctor's Dietitian*. Pork is a lean meat comparable to skinless chicken. The combination of apples and carrots with ginger and sage makes this a delightful main dish.

Serves 4

Ingredients

4 ½ boneless skinless pork loins (about ½ inch thick or 4 ounces each)
1 tablespoon of extra virgin olive oil, divided
1 teaspoon ground ginger
½ teaspoon ground sage
¼ teaspoon freshly ground black pepper
1 tablespoon unsalted butter
1 large apple (Pink Lady works well), peeled, cored and cubed
1 cup diced carrots (approximately 5 small)
¼ cup water

Instructions

Rub half the olive oil on all sides of pork. Mix ginger, sage, and pepper together and rub on both sides of pork chops.

Heat the other half of the oil in a large skillet over medium heat. Add pork to the skillet and sauté until brown, about 3 to 4 minutes per side and then transfer to a platter.

Add butter, chopped apple, and carrots to the skillet and sauté until golden brown. Stir in approximately ¼ cup of water and cook until tender. Add pork to the skillet and simmer until hot.

337 calories • 11 g carbohydrate • 2 g fiber • 6 g fat (2 g saturated fat) • 33 g protein • 90 mg sodium

Shrimp Scampi with Broccoli

Using olive oil and a little bit of butter gives this classic Italian dish a healthy makeover without sacrificing flavor. Shrimp are high in protein and omega-3 fats which can lower inflammation.

Serves 4 (makes 6 cups)

Ingredients

4 cups of cooked whole wheat fettuccini pasta
(½ pound uncooked)
2 ½ cup broccoli florets
1 tablespoon unsalted butter
2 tablespoons of good quality extra virgin olive oil
4 cloves of finely chopped garlic
1 pound shrimp, peeled and cleaned
½ cup dry white wine
⅛ teaspoon kosher salt
¼ teaspoon freshly ground pepper
1 teaspoon of grated lemon zest
Juice from ½ a lemon
Pinch of red pepper flakes

Instructions

Cook pasta according to package instructions. Two minutes before pasta is done, add broccoli.

While pasta is cooking, melt butter in a large saucepan under low heat. Add olive oil and garlic. Sauté for 2 to 3 minutes.

Add shrimp and cook on medium heat until cooked (shrimp should be pink on both sides).

Reduce heat to low. Add wine, salt, pepper, lemon zest and juice, and red pepper. Mix well. Add drained pasta and broccoli. Toss to combine then serve immediately.

Tips

► To lower the glycemic index of pasta, cook it "al dente" or at the lowest recommended cooking time.
► Resist the urge to buy pre-cleaned and cooked shrimp, which can taste dry. Instead, buy cleaned and deveined shrimp with the skin still on. Peel the skins off just before cooking.
► Grate the lemon before squeezing it for juice.

380 calories • 44 g carbohydrate • 8 g fiber • 11 g fat (3 g saturated fat) • 25 g protein • 675 mg sodium

Salmon Cakes
with Greek Yogurt Lemon Aioli

These salmon cakes provide a good source of healthy omega-3 fats and protein. Greek yogurt lemon aioli is the perfect condiment.

Serves 4

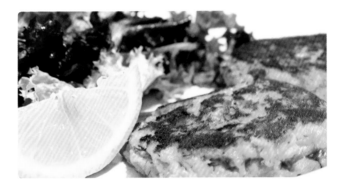

Ingredients

1, (6 ounce) can of boneless, skinless Sockeye salmon
¾ cup whole wheat bread crumbs
1 egg
2 tablespoons celery, finely chopped
1 tablespoon Dijon mustard
1 tablespoon Greek yogurt
1 teaspoon fresh dill, roughly chopped
Zest of **1** lemon
⅛ teaspoon kosher salt
¼ teaspoon freshly ground black pepper
¼ teaspoon garlic powder
1 tablespoon green onion, finely chopped (green parts only)
Cooking spray
2 tablespoons Greek Yogurt Lemon Aoli (**see next page**)
½ lemon, sliced in wedges

Instructions

In a medium sized mixing bowl combine salmon, bread crumbs, egg, celery, mustard, yogurt, dill, lemon zest, salt, pepper, garlic powder, and green onion. Use a fork to break apart salmon and mix well.

Form salmon mixture into 4 cakes, roughly ½ inch thick.

Spray a large frying pan with non-stick cooking spray and heat over medium high heat. Add cakes and cook 2 to 3 minutes on each side.

Top with Greek Yogurt Lemon Aoli and lemon wedges.

Serve immediately.

260 calories, 20 g carbohydrate, 2 g fiber, 10 g fat (2 g saturated fat), 20 g protein, 580 mg sodium

Greek Yogurt Lemon Aioli

Serves 4

Ingredients

½ cup plain Greek yogurt
1 tablespoon olive oil based
mayonnaise
Juice of half a lemon
½ teaspoon garlic powder
1 teaspoon fresh dill,
roughly chopped
⅛ teaspoon kosher salt
⅛ teaspoon freshly ground
black pepper

Instructions

Whisk all ingredients in a small
bowl. Serve immediately or chill
up to 2 days.

2 tablespoons:
30 calories • 2 g carbohydrate • 0 g fiber • 1.5 g fat (0 g saturated fat) • 3 g protein • 130 mg sodium

Pineapple Chicken Kabobs

Garlic and lemon zest provide rich flavor to this summer favorite.

Serves 4

Ingredients

5 tablespoons extra virgin olive oil, divided

3 cloves of garlic, minced

2 teaspoons lemon zest

1 tablespoon fresh parsley, chopped

½ teaspoon freshly ground black pepper

1 teaspoon kosher salt, divided

1 pound boneless, skinless chicken breast, cut into 2 inch cubes

10 ounce pineapple, cut into 1 to 2 inch pieces

1 bell pepper, cut into 1 to 2 inch pieces

½ red onion, cut into 1 to 2 inch pieces

1 yellow squash or zucchini, cut into 1 to 2 inch pieces

Juice of **1** lemon

1 cup wild rice

4 - 6 metal or wooden skewers

Instructions

In a large bowl, whisk half of the olive oil, garlic, lemon zest, parsley, pepper, and ½ teaspoon of salt. Add chicken and mix well.

In a small bowl whisk together remaining olive oil, salt, and lemon juice. Set aside.

Heat grill on medium-high heat.

Thread chicken, pineapple, and vegetables on skewers in a varied pattern. Brush kabobs with lemon juice and olive oil mixture. Add kabobs to grill and cook 8 to 12 minutes or until chicken is cooked throughout or reaches an internal temperature of 165°F.

While kabobs are grilling, cook rice according to package directions.

Remove kabobs from grill and serve over rice.

Tips

▸ Add other vegetables like mushrooms for variety.
▸ Shrimp is a good substitute for chicken.

400 calories • 37 g carbohydrate • 2 g fiber • 17 g fat (2.5 g saturated fat) • 24 g protein • 510 mg sodium

Spaghetti Squash and Meatballs

This meal is a substitute for the Italian classic spaghetti and meatballs with significantly less carbohydrates and fat. Spaghetti squash is a good source of fiber and vitamin A.

Serves 4

Ingredients

1 large spaghetti squash cut in half
¼ cup water
4 cups low sodium, low sugar prepared marinara sauce
12 meatballs (recipe below)
⅛ teaspoon kosher salt
¼ teaspoon freshly ground black pepper
1 tablespoon extra virgin olive oil
4 fresh basil leaves, roughly chopped (garnish)

Instructions

Place squash in a large microwave safe dish, cut side up. Pour water in the bottom of the dish. Cover tightly with plastic wrap. Microwave on high for 15 to 18 minutes.

While squash is cooking, heat sauce and meatballs over medium-low heat in a large sauce pan.

When squash is cooked, remove from dish and let sit 5 minutes. Scoop out the inside of squash into a large bowl. Add, salt, pepper, and olive oil. Lightly mix.

Divide squash among plates and top with marinara and meatballs. Garnish with fresh basil.

(see meatball recipe on next page)

470 calories • 30 g carbohydrate • 5 g fiber • 23 g fat (4 g saturated fat) • 33 g protein • 560 mg sodium

Meatballs

Makes 12 meatballs

Ingredients

1 pound 93% lean ground beef
½ pound ground chicken
¾ cup panko bread crumbs
2 eggs
½ teaspoon garlic powder
½ teaspoon fennel seed
¼ teaspoon kosher salt
¼ teaspoon freshly ground
   black pepper
1 tablespoon fresh parsley,
   chopped

Instructions

Preheat oven to 350°F.

Combine all ingredients in a
large mixing bowl. Mix well with
hands to evenly combine.

Roll mixture into balls, 2 inches
in diameter. Place on a large
cookie sheet. Bake until browned,
approximately 12 minutes.

Tip
▸ Prepared, these meatballs freeze well for leftovers.

3 meatballs:
280 calories, 16 g carbohydrate, <1 g fiber, 10 g fat (3.5 g saturated fat), 30 g protein, 400 mg sodium

Italian Polenta Casserole

Most casseroles are made with canned soups or unhealthy
ingredients. This easy dish uses fresh vegetables
and chicken sausage for a healthier version.

Serves 5

Ingredients

1, (18 ounce) tube of pre-cooked
packaged polenta

2 tablespoons extra virgin
olive oil, divided

1 small white onion, diced

3 cloves garlic, minced

3 Italian-Style chicken sausage
links, casings removed

1 large zucchini, cut in 1
inch pieces

1, (28 ounce) can fire roasted
diced tomatoes

1 ½ cups frozen chopped spinach,
thawed

½ teaspoon freshly ground
black pepper

¼ teaspoon crushed red pepper

1 cup shredded part-skim, low
sodium mozzarella cheese

Instructions

Preheat oven to 375°F.

Slice polenta in ½ inch rounds.
Brush both sides of polenta
rounds with 1 tablespoon of olive
oil. Place rounds in bottom of a
medium casserole dish. Cover as
much of the bottom of the dish as
possible. It may be necessary
to cut rounds in half to make
them fit better. Bake polenta in
oven for 20 minutes.

While polenta is cooking, heat
remaining oil in a large sauté
pan over medium heat. Add onions and sauté until just soft. Add
garlic and sauté 1 minute.

Add sausage links to sauté pan.
Break pieces with spoon as you
sauté. Once sausage starts to
brown add zucchini, tomatoes,
spinach, pepper, and crushed
red pepper.

Instructions

Continue to cook until zucchini is softened.

Using a slotted spoon, top polenta with sausage and vegetable mixture. Sprinkle with mozzarella cheese and return casserole dish to oven.

Bake 10 to 15 minutes or until bubbling.

Allow dish to sit 10 to15 minutes before serving.

Tip

▸ This dish reheats well. Store in refrigerator for up to 3 days or freeze until you are ready to reheat.

280 calories • 20 g carbohydrate • 1 g fiber • 14 g fat (5 g saturated fat) • 18 g protein • 580 mg sodium

Grilled Salmon with Pineapple Mango Salsa

No salty marinade needed for this delicious dish! Freshly cut pineapple and mango give omega-3 rich salmon a sweet and juicy topping.

Serves 4 fillets

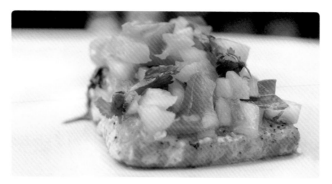

Ingredients

4, 6 ounce skinless salmon filets
3 tablespoons extra virgin olive oil
½ teaspoon kosher salt
½ teaspoon freshly ground pepper
½ cup Pineapple Mango Salsa

Instructions

Preheat grill or grill pan. Prepare the salmon by brushing on oil. Sprinkle with salt and pepper.

Grill the salmon over direct heat on the first side, about 6 to 7 minutes. Turn fish and cook on the second side, about 5 to 6 minutes. Fish should be opaque or reach an internal temperature of 140°F.

Top each fillet with ½ cup salsa.

Serve immediately.

(see salsa recipe on next page)

Tip

▸ If using a barbeque, a grill pan will allow you to easily turn the fish and prevent it from breaking apart.

440 calories, 14 g carbohydrate, 2 g fiber, 27 g fat (4 g saturated fat), 35 g protein, 368 mg sodium

Pineapple Mango Salsa

Makes 2 cups

Ingredients

1 cup chopped mango
1 cup chopped pineapple
¼ cup chopped red onion
2 tablespoons fresh lime juice
½ cup finely chopped cilantro
½ cup chopped red pepper
⅓ cup good quality extra
   virgin olive oil

Instructions

In a medium bowl combine mango, pineapple, onion, lime juice, cilantro, red pepper and oil. Mix well.

Tips

▸ To avoid the salsa from getting too watery, cut the pineapple first and place it in a separate bowl. Then drain extra juice.
▸ Refrigerate the prepared salsa for 30 minutes or up to a day before using to intensify the flavor.
▸ Double the recipe for extra salsa to put over other fish dishes or on the Black Bean Cakes.

½ cup:
198 calories, 14 g carbohydrate, 2 g fiber, 17 g fat (2 g saturated fat), 1 g protein, 2 mg sodium

Grilled Chicken Thighs

This savory recipe is shared by Dr. Stephanie Mattei from the
Center for Acceptance and Change and co-author of
**The PCOS Workbook: Your Guide to Complete
Physical and Emotional Health.**

Serves 4

Ingredients

8 skinless, boneless chicken
thighs (about 2 pounds)
2 teaspoons dried parsley
1 teaspoon dried basil
½ teaspoon freshly ground
black pepper
½ teaspoon seasoned salt
½ teaspoon onion powder
2 tablespoons extra virgin
olive oil

Instructions

Rinse chicken under cold water,
and pat dry with paper towels.

Place the chicken thighs in a
wide flat dish so they are in a
single layer. Add parsley, basil,
pepper, salt, onion powder, and
oil. Rub the thighs to coat with
the herb mixture. Cover and
refrigerate up to 24 hours.

Note: If doing a quick marinade,
leave the chicken out of the
refrigerator for up to 1 hour.

Preheat grill on medium heat.

Remove chicken from dish
and discard marinade. Place
chicken on the grill and cook
until done or reaches an
internal temperature of 165°F
(about 8 to 10 minutes
each side).

439 calories • 0 g carbohydrate • 0 g fiber • 22 g fat (5 g saturated fat) • 57 g protein, 461 mg sodium

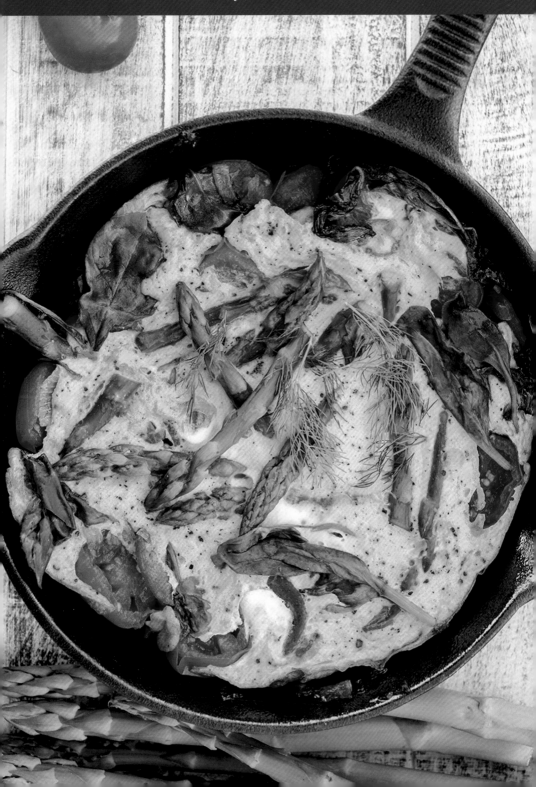

Broccoli and Cheddar Crustless Quiche

This quiche is so tasty you won't miss the crust or the carbohydrates.

Serves 5

Ingredients

1 tablespoon canola oil
½ onion, roughly chopped
Cooking spray
1 small head broccoli, stemmed
   and cut into small florets
2 cups extra sharp cheddar
   cheese, shredded
2 tablespoons quinoa flour
6 eggs
⅓ cup 1% milk
¼ teaspoon kosher salt
¼ teaspoon freshly
   ground black pepper
¼ teaspoon garlic powder
1 cup kale, chopped

Instructions

Preheat oven to 350°F.

Heat oil in a small skillet over medium heat. Add onions and sauté until browned, about 10 minutes.

Coat an 8-inch glass pie plate with cooking spray. Place onions in the bottom. Spread broccoli florets over top.

In a small bowl mix cheese and quinoa flour. Sprinkle over top of broccoli and onions.

In a medium bowl, beat together eggs, milk, salt, pepper, and garlic powder. Pour over broccoli and cheese. Sprinkle kale over top. Bake in oven for 25 minutes or until set in center and golden brown at edges.

Serve immediately.

Tip

▸ Buy pre-chopped kale and portion it into smaller freezer bags. Store kale in freezer for casseroles and smoothies.

270 calories • 14 g carbohydrate • 4 g fiber • 17 g fat (7 g saturated fat) • 18 g protein • 390 mg sodium

Garden Herb Quinoa, Chickpea and Arugula Salad

This salad is full of flavor and fiber. Fiber is important for helping control blood sugar levels by slowing the release of glucose into the blood stream.

Serves 4

Ingredients

½ cup quinoa, dry
1 teaspoon canola oil
1 small onion, thinly sliced
⅛ teaspoon kosher salt
1 teaspoon cumin
½ cup Italian flat leaf parsley, roughly chopped
2 tablespoons fresh mint, roughly chopped
1 tablespoon fresh basil, roughly chopped
2 tablespoons lemon juice
¼ cup extra virgin olive oil
2 green onions, diced
⅓ cup golden raisins
½ cup slivered almonds
½ cup feta cheese, crumbled
1 teaspoon lemon zest
1, (15 ounce) can chickpeas, rinsed and drained
¼ teaspoon freshly ground black pepper
4 cups arugula

Instructions

Cook quinoa according to package instructions. Fluff with fork. Set aside to cool.

Heat canola oil in a medium sized frying pan over medium-high heat. Add onions, salt, and cumin. Sauté until caramelized, about 10 to 12 minutes. Once onions are cooked, remove from heat and set aside to cool.

While onions are cooking, add parsley, mint, basil, lemon juice, and olive oil in food processor. Process 30 seconds. Set aside.

In a large bowl add green onion, raisins, almonds, feta, lemon zest, chickpeas, and quinoa. Pour herb mixture over top, add black pepper, and mix well.

Fold in arugula. Divide salad on 4 plates and top each salad with caramelized onions.

Serve immediately.

Tip

▸ For leftovers the next day, only add arugula to half of the quinoa and herb mixture. Pack arugula separately and combine when you're ready to eat to avoid soggy leaves.

440 calories • 46 g carbohydrate • 9 g fiber • 21 g fat (5 g saturated fat) • 15 g protein • 390 mg sodium

Cauliflower Crust Pizza

If pizza normally leaves you feeling like you overindulged, you'll love this version with a crispy cauliflower crust. Over 100% of the recommended amounts for vitamins A and C are found in one serving of this tasty pie.

Serves 3

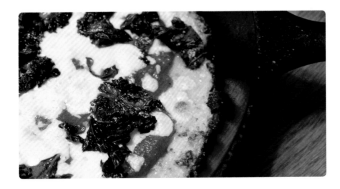

Ingredients

1 small head of cauliflower, cut into florets
½ cup almond flour
⅓ cup shredded cheddar cheese
1 tablespoon grated parmesan cheese
½ teaspoon dried oregano
¼ teaspoon dried basil
¼ teaspoon garlic powder
¼ teaspoon black pepper
¼ teaspoon salt, divided
2 eggs
Cooking spray
1 teaspoon canola oil
2 cups kale, chopped
⅛ teaspoon crushed red pepper
1 cup prepared pizza sauce
4 ounces shredded mozzarella cheese

Instructions

Preheat oven to 450°F.

Place a medium sized cast iron skillet in oven while it heats.

Pulse cauliflower florets in a food processor until it resembles rice. Measure 3 ½ cups of the riced cauliflower. Place in a microwave safe bowl and cook on high for 6 to 7 minutes. Remove from bowl and wrap in paper towels, pressing to remove excess water. Allow to cool 5 to 10 minutes.

In a large bowl, mix cauliflower, almond flour, cheddar and parmesan cheeses, oregano, basil, garlic powder, black pepper, half of salt, and eggs to form a dough.

Remove skillet from oven and spray with cooking spray. Press dough into bottom of skillet. Bake 15 minutes or until crust is golden brown. Remove from oven.

While crust is cooking, heat oil in a medium sauté pan over medium heat. Add kale and season with remaining salt and crushed red pepper. Sauté 5 minutes or until leaves have softened. Set aside.

Top crust with sauce, leaving 1 inch uncovered at edges. Top with mozzarella and kale. Return to oven and cook 10 more minutes or until cheese is bubbling. Allow to cool slightly before serving.

Tips

- Add chopped fresh basil to your sauce to add extra flavor.
- Remaining riced cauliflower can be refrigerated up to 2 days and used in other recipes, such as the Slow-Cooker Stuffed Peppers.

270 calories, 21 g carbohydrate, 8 g fiber, 20 g fat (8 g saturated fat), 25 g protein, 580 mg sodium

Natalie's
Cauliflower Fried "Rice"

Fried rice is typically high in carbohydrates and sodium.
This version of the take-out classic cuts both of these in half and adds
a healthy serving of veggies! It's so tasty, you won't miss the real deal.

Serves 4

Ingredients

1 head of cauliflower,
　　cut into florets
2 tablespoons canola oil,
　　divided
1 small onion, diced
3 cloves garlic, minced
1 tablespoon minced ginger
1 ½ cups mushrooms, diced
1 zucchini, cut in one inch
　　pieces (about **1 ½** cups)
1 cup shredded carrots
3 tablespoons low sodium
　　tamari or soy sauce, divided
½ cup unsalted cashews
1 green onion, diced
3 eggs, lightly beaten
1 teaspoon sesame oil

Instructions

Using the grating attachment
on your food processor, grate
cauliflower florets. This should
yield approximately 7 cups.
Set aside.

Heat one tablespoon of
canola oil in a medium skillet
over medium-high heat. Add
onion, garlic, and ginger. Cook
until fragrant, about 2 minutes.
Add mushrooms, zucchini, and
carrots. Sauté 5 minutes or until
vegetables are just tender.
Add 1 tablespoon tamari,
cashews, and green onion.
Remove from heat and
set aside.

In a large wok or skillet, heat
remaining oil over medium-high
heat. Add riced cauliflower.
Sauté 1 to 2 minutes. Using a
spoon, create a well in the
center of the pan. Add egg
and scramble, incorporating
it into rice.

Add sautéed vegetables,
remaining tamari, and sesame
oil. Sauté 1 to 2 minutes, or until
heated through.

Tip

► If you don't have a grater attachment for your food processor, you can pulse the cauliflower in the processor. Grating the cauliflower makes this dish a little fluffier and more authentic.

320 calories •27 g carbohydrate •8 g fiber •20 g fat (3.5 g saturated fat) •14 g protein •530 mg sodium

Broccoli and Tempeh with Garlic Sauce

The typical broccoli and garlic sauce dish is loaded with sodium and additives. Our version reduces the sodium, but adds protein without losing flavor. Tempeh, fermented soy, is high in protein.

Serves 3

Ingredients

1 cup cooked brown rice
3 cloves of garlic, minced
1 tablespoon fresh ginger, minced
1 tablespoon chili garlic sauce
2 tablespoons low sodium tamari or soy sauce
⅓ cup low sodium vegetable broth
¼ cup water
1 tablespoon pure maple syrup
1, (8 ounce) package tempeh
1 large head broccoli, trimmed into florets
1 cup chopped asparagus
2 teaspoons cornstarch dissolved in **2** tablespoons water

Instructions

In a large frying pan or wok combine garlic, ginger, chili garlic sauce, soy sauce, broth, water, and maple syrup. Stir and heat over medium-high heat. Bring to boil and cook 5 minutes.

Add tempeh, broccoli, asparagus, and dissolved cornstarch. Cook 10 minutes over medium heat or until vegetables are tender.

Remove from heat and serve over brown rice.

Tips

▸ You can find chili garlic sauce in the Asian or international section of the grocery store.
▸ Use instant microwavable rice to save time.

290 calories • 45 g carbohydrate • 9 g fiber • 5 g fat (1 g saturated fat • 19 g protein • 400 mg sodium

Tomato and Lentil Vinaigrette Salad

Members of the legume family, lentils are high in fiber and protein. Unlike beans, lentils don't need pre-soaking. Enjoy this tasty salad as a warm side dish to fish, meat, or poultry, or on its own as a main dish.

Serves 4

Ingredients

4 cups water
1 ¼ cup dried lentils, rinsed
1 cup chopped carrot
⅓ cup chopped onion
1 tablespoon finely
   chopped garlic
1 bay leaf
¼ cup red wine vinegar
2 cups of grape tomatoes,
   cut in half
½ teaspoon kosher salt
½ teaspoon freshly
   ground pepper
¼ cup chopped fresh parsley

Instructions

In a large saucepan, combine water, lentils, carrot, onion, garlic and bay leaf. Cook over high heat, stirring occasionally until mixture reaches a full boil.

Reduce heat to low. Cover and cook until lentils are tender (about 25 to 35 minutes), stirring occasionally. Drain lentils and discard bay leaf.

In a large bowl, combine warm lentil mixture, red wine vinegar, tomatoes, salt, pepper, and parsley. Toss to coat well.

Serve warm or cold.

97 calories • 18 g carbohydrate • 6 g fiber • < 1 g fat (< 1 g saturated fat) • 6 g protein • 456 mg sodium

Japanese Eggplant and Mushroom Stir-Fry with Seitan

Here's a protein rich stir-fry that's so tasty, you won't miss the meat! Seitan (pronounced "say-tan"), also known as wheat gluten, is high in protein and low in fat with a meaty texture.

Serves 4

Ingredients

- 1 ¾ cups water
- 1 cup brown rice, uncooked
- 3 Japanese eggplants, diced into 2 inch pieces
- ⅛ teaspoon kosher salt
- 2 tablespoons sambal oelek (garlic chili paste)
- 1 teaspoon paprika
- 1 teaspoon Mexican style chili powder
- 3 tablespoons canola oil, divided
- 3 cloves of garlic, diced
- 1 tablespoon fresh ginger, minced
- 2 scallions, diced (green and white parts)
- 1, (3.5 ounce) container shiitake mushrooms, stemmed and sliced
- 1, (8 ounce) container baby Portobello mushrooms, sliced
- 1, (20 ounce) container cubed seitan, drained
- 1 tablespoon Bragg liquid amino acids
- 2 tablespoons balsamic vinegar

Instructions

In a small sauce pan, combine water and rice. Bring to a boil, cover and reduce to a simmer. Cook 45 minutes, or until rice has absorbed water. Set aside.

Place eggplant slices in colander and toss with salt. Set aside.

In a small bowl, whisk together sambal oelek, paprika, and chili powder to form a paste. Set aside.

In a large wok or sauté pan, heat half of canola oil over medium-high heat. Add garlic, ginger, and scallions. Sauté until fragrant, about 2 to 3 minutes. Add eggplant and sauté until just tender, about 5 to 8 minutes. Add remaining oil, mushrooms, and seitan. Mix well. Add spice paste. Sauté 10 minutes or until mushrooms are softened, stirring often. Add amino acids and balsamic vinegar. Mix well.

Remove from heat and serve over brown rice.

Tip

▸ You can find sambal oelek in the Asian or international
section of the grocery store.
▸ To save time, use precooked brown rice.

330 calories • 40 g carbohydrate • 6 g fiber • 13 g fat (1 g saturated fat) • 16 g protein • 420 mg sodium

Super-Fast
Soba Noodle Salad

This tasty salad takes very little time to make and packs
well for a healthy lunch. Soba noodles are high in fiber.
Red cabbage and sesame seeds add crunch to every bite.

Serves 5

Ingredients

1, (8 ounce) package
   buckwheat soba noodles
2 cups cucumber, diced
2 cups red cabbage, chopped
2 green onions, chopped
   (white and green parts)
1 ½ cups frozen edamame,
   unthawed
¼ cup sesame seeds
½ cup chopped cilantro
2 tablespoons sesame oil
2 tablespoons low sodium
   tamari or soy sauce
4 tablespoons balsamic vinegar
1 tablespoon pure maple syrup

Instructions

Cook soba noodles according
to package instructions. Drain
and rinse with cold water.

In a large bowl combine cooked
noodles, cucumber, red cabbage, green onions, edamame,
sesame seeds, and cilantro.

In a small bowl, whisk together
sesame oil, tamari, balsamic
vinegar, and maple syrup.

Pour vinaigrette over noodles
and vegetables. Toss well to
combine.

Serve at room temperature or
chill. Refrigerate in an airtight
container for up to 3 days.

Tip

► To cut down on prep time, look for pre-packaged diced
   red cabbage.

340 calories • 45 g carbohydrate • 5 g fiber • 14 g fat (1.5 g saturated fat) • 14 g protein • 560 mg sodium

Tempeh Teriyaki Stir-Fry

Tempeh, a fermented soy product, is a natural probiotic which can help with digestion and inflammation. Our homemade teriyaki sauce is lower in sodium and has no preservatives or artificial flavors compared to a bottled brand-and much tastier!

Serves 2

Ingredients

Tempeh Stir-Fry:
1 tablespoon coconut oil
  plus 1 teaspoon
8 ounces of tempeh, cut
  into cubes
2 ½ cups broccoli florets
1 ½ cups chopped carrots
1 cup snow peas
1 cup cooked brown rice
⅓ cup unsalted cashew halves

Teriyaki Sauce:
2 tablespoons low-sodium
  soy sauce
1 teaspoon honey
1 tablespoon peeled,
  grated fresh ginger

Instructions

Heat 1 tablespoon of coconut oil in a large non-stick skillet or wok over medium heat until melted. Add tempeh and cook over medium-high heat until golden brown on all sides, turning occasionally. Transfer tempeh to a plate lined with a paper towel. Set aside.

Heat remaining coconut oil. Add broccoli, carrots, and snow peas. Cook over medium-high heat, stirring constantly until vegetables are tender but still crisp. Reduce heat to low.

To make teriyaki sauce, whisk together soy sauce and honey in a small saucepan over low heat. Bring to a simmer. Add ginger and stir. Remove from heat.

Add tempeh and sauce to vegetables and mix well. Add rice and cashews and stir to combine.

Tip
▸ Any type of vegetable works well with this dish, so toss in your favorites.

560 calories • 57 g carbohydrate • 17 g fiber • 26 g fat (11 g saturated fat) • 31 g protein • 451 mg sodium

Peanut Noodles with Tofu and Broccoli

This meal combines the delightful flavors of ginger, honey, sesame, and peanuts. High in fiber and protein, this dish will satisfy you and your taste buds.

Serves 4

Ingredients

Cooking spray
1 tablespoon extra virgin olive oil, divided
1 teaspoon low sodium tamari or soy sauce plus 1 tablespoon
1, (14 ounce) package extra firm tofu, pressed and cut into 1 inch cubes
6 ounces soba noodles (two wrapped bundles)
2 cloves garlic, minced
2 tablespoons fresh ginger, minced
1 ½ cups water
1 teaspoon honey
1 tablespoon peanut butter
1 teaspoon sesame oil
4 cups frozen broccoli florets, thawed
¼ cup cilantro, roughly chopped
2 scallions (green parts only), diced
¼ cup dry roasted, unsalted peanuts, chopped

Instructions

Preheat oven to 375°F.

Coat baking sheet with cooking spray.

In a small bowl, whisk half of the olive oil and teaspoon of tamari. Brush mixture over tofu. Place tofu on baking sheet. Bake 15 minutes, then flip. Return to oven for an additional 15 minutes.

Prepare soba noodles according to package directions. Set aside.

In a large sauce pan, heat remaining olive oil over medium heat. Add garlic and ginger. Sauté until just fragrant, about 1 to 2 minutes. Whisk in remaining tablespoon of tamari, water, honey, peanut butter, and sesame oil. Heat until sauce just begins to boil.

Instructions

Once sauce begins to boil, add soba noodles and broccoli. Add cilantro and toss well to coat noodles.

Serve noodles in bowls. Top each bowl with ¼ of the baked tofu and garnish with scallions and peanuts.

Serve immediately.

Tips

- Other vegetables such as mushrooms or zucchini can be added increase the nutrient value of this dish.
- We recommend purchasing non-GMO tofu brands.

430 calories • 51 g carbohydrate • 8 g fiber • 17 g fat (2 g saturated fat) • 29 g protein • 590 mg sodium

Falafels with Cucumber Dill Sauce

A Middle Eastern favorite! Meatless and low GI, this satisfying dish uses significantly less oil than the traditional deep-fried version.

Serves 4 (makes 8 falafels)

Ingredients

Falafels

- **1** (15.5 ounce) can of garbanzo beans (chickpeas), rinsed and drained
- **1** cup chopped yellow onion
- **3** cloves garlic, peeled
- **1** large egg, slightly beaten
- **1** teaspoon baking powder
- **1** teaspoon ground cumin
- **1** teaspoon ground coriander
- **¼** teaspoon kosher salt
- **¼** teaspoon freshly ground pepper
- **¼** cup chopped parsley
- **1** teaspoon freshly squeezed lemon juice
- **⅓** cup fava bean flour plus **2** tablespoons
- **1** tablespoon canola oil

Cucumber Dill Sauce

Makes 1 cup

- **1** (6 ounce) container plain Greek yogurt
- **1** teaspoon freshly squeezed lemon juice
- **1** tablespoon freshly chopped dill
- **1** clove garlic, peeled
- **½** cucumber, peeled and diced

Instructions

To make falafels, place chickpeas in a large bowl and mash with fork.

Place onion and garlic in a food processor. Process until smooth. Add to chickpeas. Add egg, baking powder, cumin, coriander, salt, pepper, parsley, lemon juice, and ⅓ cup flour. Mix well.

Place remaining flour on a large plate. Form chickpea mixture into 8 balls. Roll each ball into flour, pressing down to form a patty.

To make the cucumber dill sauce, place all ingredients in food processor. Process until well combined. Store in a covered bowl in the refrigerator until ready to use.

Instructions

Heat oil in a 10 inch cast iron skillet over medium heat. Place patties on skillet and cook until golden brown and crispy, about 3 minutes each side. Top each falafel with 1 tablespoon cucumber dill sauce and serve.

Tip

 ▸ Purchased tzatziki sauce can be a quick alternative to preparing the cucumber dill sauce.

239 calories • 31 g carbohydrate • 9 g fiber • 7 g fat (1 g saturated fat) • 16 g protein • 316 mg sodium

Garden Frittata

This one pot meal is an easy weeknight dinner that's doesn't skimp on protein and veggies. Freshly chopped herbs provide a delicate bite.

Serves 4

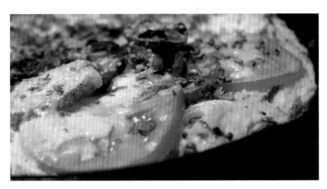

Ingredients

2 tablespoons extra virgin olive oil
2 cups asparagus, cut into
    1 inch pieces
3 small red potatoes, sliced
1 small shallot, diced
8 eggs
¼ cup lowfat milk
¼ teaspoon kosher salt
¼ teaspoon freshly ground
    black pepper
1 tomato, cut into ¼ inch slices
¼ cup ricotta salata cheese,
    crumbled
1 tablespoon fresh parsley,
    chopped
1 tablespoon chives, chopped

Instructions

Preheat oven to 500°F.

Heat oil in a medium cast iron or oven safe skillet over medium heat. Add asparagus, potatoes, and shallot. Sauté until brown spots start to appear on potatoes. Set aside ½ cup of vegetables.

Combine eggs with milk, salt, and pepper. Beat well. Add to hot skillet with sautéed vegetables. Continue to cook over medium heat. Push eggs with spatula from edges to the center of the pan until eggs are almost cooked.

Instructions

Remove from heat. Top egg mixture with remaining vegetables, tomato slices, and cheese. Place in oven for 3-5 minutes.

Remove from oven and sprinkle with chopped parsley and chives.

Tip

 Don't scramble the eggs. Just push them deliberately around the pan.

310 calories • 17 g carbohydrate • 4 g fiber • 18 g fat (5 g saturated fat) • 19 g protein • 410 mg sodium

Black Bean Cakes

A favorite recipe among our patients with PCOS, these black bean cakes make a tasty and filling meatless meal. Low GI black beans provide protein and iron. If you aren't familiar with panko, they are Japanese bread crumbs.

Serves 4

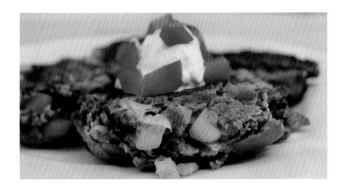

Ingredients

2 tablespoons extra virgin olive oil
½ cup finely chopped yellow onion
2 cloves minced garlic
¼ cup chopped red pepper
½ teaspoon ground cumin
½ teaspoon ground coriander
½ teaspoon kosher salt
¼ teaspoon freshly ground pepper
1 (15.5 ounce) can black beans, rinsed and drained
2 large eggs, lightly beaten
¼ cup sliced green onions
½ cup whole wheat panko
2 tablespoons finely chopped cilantro
4 tablespoons sour cream

Instructions

Heat 1 tablespoon of oil in a medium skillet over medium heat. Add onions, garlic, and red pepper. Cook until soft, about 4 minutes, stirring occasionally. Stir in cumin, coriander, salt, and pepper. Remove from heat.

Place beans in medium bowl; coarsely mash with fork. Stir in eggs. Stir in onion mixture. Add green onions and panko and mix well. Stir in cilantro. Refrigerate for 15 to 30 minutes.

Instructions

Divide bean mixture into 4 portions, shaping each into a ½-inch thick patty. Heat a non-stick skillet over medium heat. Add remaining 1 tablespoon oil. Add patties to pan. Cook on each side until brown, about 3 minutes.

Top each black bean cake with 1 tablespoon of sour cream.

Tip

▸ The Mango Pineapple Salsa recipe is a delicious alternative to sour cream.
▸ Black bean cakes can be made and frozen for a quick reheatable lunch or dinner.
▸ To make these gluten-free, substitute gluten-free bread crumbs or almond flour for panko.

361 calories • 30 g carbohydrate • 6 g fiber • 22 g fat (4 g saturated fat) • 12 g protein • 316 mg sodium

Mini Quinoa Kale Quiches

This recipe is our cookbook contest winner! We chose it because of its taste, creativity, ease, and versatility-these mini quiches can be a healthy snack, small breakfast when paired with fruit, an appetizer, or a side dish. Thanks to Maiah Miller for her submission.

Serves 12

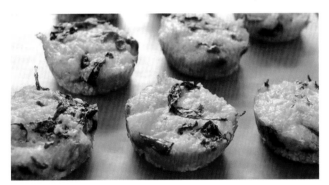

Ingredients

Cooking spray
½ cup quinoa
1 cup water
2 tablespoons extra virgin
    olive oil
1 bunch kale, stems removed
and cut into strips
1 cup mushrooms, thinly sliced
½ medium onion (about 1 cup),
    diced
2 cloves of garlic, minced
4 large eggs, beaten
½ teaspoon kosher salt
¾ teaspoon freshly ground
    black pepper

Instructions

Preheat the oven to 400°F. Spray a muffin pan with cooking spray.

Combine the quinoa and water in a small pan. Bring to a boil on medium-high and then reduce to a simmer until the water is absorbed, about 15 minutes. Set aside.

In a large sauté pan, caramelize the mushrooms and onions in the olive oil over medium heat. Cook until onion is soft and lightly browned, about 10 minutes, stirring occasionally. Place the mushrooms and onions in a large mixing bowl.

Instructions

Add kale into the previously used hot pan. Over medium heat, cook the kale until it's wilted and bright green, about two minutes. Allow kale to cool. Squeeze any extra liquid out using a paper towel or clean dish towel. Add the kale, quinoa, and garlic to the mixing bowl. Stir until combined. Pour the eggs over the quinoa and kale mixture. Add salt and pepper. Mix well.

Pour the mixture into the tin filling each cup about 7/8 full. Bake for about 15 minutes, or until the top is golden and the mixture has started to pull away from the edges of the cup. Cool 2-3 minutes on a wire rack and enjoy warm.

Tip

▸ These freeze and reheat well. Consider doubling the recipe to make extras to use as snacks.

60 calories • 5 g carbohydrate • 1 g fiber • 3 g fat (< 1 g saturated fat) • 2 g protein • 114 mg sodium

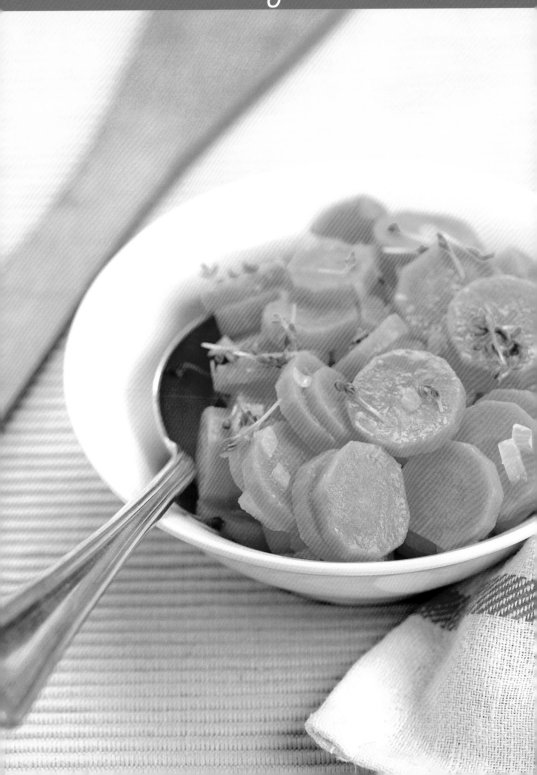

Roasted Brussels Sprouts Medley

Looking for an alternative to steamed vegetables? Try roasting them. These veggies are so flavorful they'll be a welcome addition to your dinner plate.

Serves 4

Ingredients

- ¼ pound Brussels sprouts, halved
- 1 fennel bulb, cut into thin wedges (green parts removed)
- 2 cups cauliflower florets
- 3 tablespoons extra virgin olive oil, divided
- ½ teaspoon freshly ground black pepper
- ¼ teaspoon kosher salt
- 1 small head of radicchio, cored and cut into thin wedges.

Instructions

Preheat oven to 400°F.

Place Brussels sprouts, fennel, and cauliflower on a large baking sheet. Drizzle with half of oil and season with salt and pepper. Lightly toss vegetables to coat evenly. Roast in oven for 15 minutes.

Remove from vegetables from oven. Add radicchio and drizzle with remaining olive oil. Return to oven and roast an additional 15 minutes or until all vegetables begin to caramelize and brown on edges.

Serve immediately.

Tip

▸ Different types of vegetables such as asparagus, squash, and peppers can be roasted this way as well.

130 calories • 9 g carbohydrate • 4 g fiber • 10 g fat (1 g saturated fat) • 3 g protein • 190 mg sodium

Citrus-Glazed Carrots

These carrots make a quick and sweet side dish.

Serves 4

Ingredients

1 pound of baby or
   chopped carrots
1 teaspoon of grated orange
   zest (about **1** large orange)
½ cup freshly squeezed
   orange juice
2 tablespoons unsalted butter
1 tablespoon honey
2 teaspoons fresh rosemary

Instructions

In a medium skillet combine carrots, zest, juice, butter and honey. Cover and cook until carrots are tender and most of juice is absorbed, about 10 minutes; stir occasionally. Add rosemary and mix well. Serve hot.

111 calories • 18 g carbohydrate • 3 g fiber • 4 g fat (2 g saturated fat) • 2 g protein • 81 mg sodium

Asian Slaw

This crunchy vegetable side dish provides an Asian inspired flair to coleslaw. It can be made in minutes and provides a good source of omega-3 fats. Sesame oil has antibacterial, antiviral and antifungal properties.

Serves 6

Ingredients

Asian Slaw:
10 ounce package shredded broccoli and carrot slaw
2 cups shredded cabbage
4 green onions, chopped
⅓ cup sliced almonds
½ cup sunflower seeds
1 cup cooked edamame, cooled

Dressing:
¼ cup rice wine vinegar
2 tablespoons low sodium soy sauce
½ cup toasted sesame oil
1 tablespoon honey
½ cup chopped cilantro

Instructions

In a large bowl, combine broccoli carrot slaw, cabbage, green onions, almonds, sunflower seeds, and endamame.

In a small bowl, whisk together rice wine vinegar, soy sauce, sesame oil, and honey.

Pour dressing over slaw and mix well. Add cilantro and toss to combine.

Tip

▸ To make this recipe even quicker, buy already chopped onions and shredded cabbage.

250 calories • 13 g carbohydrate • 3 g fiber • 20 g fat (3 g saturated fat) • 4 g protein • 149 mg sodium

Black Bean and Toasted Corn Salad

This easy salad is full of fiber and heart healthy fats.
It's a great addition to a meal and makes a tasty side dish for entertaining.

Serves 4

Ingredients

1 cup frozen corn, unthawed
1, (15 ounce) can black beans, rinsed and drained
1 red bell pepper, diced
1 avocado, diced
2 tablespoons diced red onion
¼ cup cilantro, finely chopped
Juice and zest of **1** lime
1 tablespoon extra virgin olive oil
¼ teaspoon kosher salt
⅛ teaspoon ground cayenne pepper
½ teaspoon freshly ground black pepper
1 teaspoon honey

Instructions

Heat a nonstick frying pan over medium heat. Add frozen corn and toast until the kernels start to brown, about 5 minutes. Set aside and cool.

In a large bowl combine beans, bell pepper, avocado, onion, cilantro, lime juice, and zest. Mix in cooled corn.

Add olive oil, salt, pepper, cayenne, and honey. Toss well.

Serve immediately or chill for later use.

Tips

▸ This salad is delicious with grilled corn cut off of the cob.
▸ Adjust the spiciness of this salad by reducing or adding cayenne pepper.
▸ To serve this salad the next day, prepare the salad without avocado and refrigerate overnight. Toss in the avocado right before serving.

240 calories • 32 g carbohydrate • 10 g fiber • 9 g fat (1.5 g saturated fat) • 8 g protein • 280 mg sodium

Quinoa with Peppers, Walnuts and Goat Cheese

Quinoa is a versatile whole grain that is rich in protein. The flavorful combination of peppers and raspberry vinaigrette gives this dish a sweet taste. Walnuts add crunch to balance the creaminess of goat cheese. It can be enjoyed warm or cold.

Serves 4

Ingredients

½ cup quinoa, uncooked
½ cup chopped yellow pepper
½ cup chopped orange pepper
⅓ cup chopped walnuts
2 tablespoons lite raspberry
   vinaigrette dressing
   (such as Annie's Naturals)
2 tablespoons goat cheese

Instructions

Rinse quinoa in a fine mesh colander under running water, scrubbing it between your hands to remove its bitter outer coating. Cook quinoa according to package instructions.

Fluff cooked quinoa with fork. Transfer to a medium serving bowl. Add yellow and orange peppers, walnuts, and goat cheese to quinoa. Add raspberry vinaigrette dressing and combine.

Serve warm or cold.

188 calories • 14 g carbohydrate • 3 g fiber • 14 g fat (7 g saturated fat) • 7 g protein • 77 mg sodium

Roasted Garlic Mashed Cauliflower

A delicious substitute to mashed potatoes, this mashed cauliflower version will soon be your new favorite side dish.

Serves 3

Ingredients

1 head of cauliflower,
   cut into florets (about 4 cups)
6 cloves of garlic, quartered
1 tablespoon extra virgin olive oil
¼ teaspoon freshly ground
   black pepper
⅛ teaspoon kosher salt
1 tablespoon cream cheese
1 tablespoon chives,
   finely chopped

Instructions

Preheat oven to 350°F.

Place a large piece of aluminum foil over baking sheet. Place cauliflower florets and garlic on top of foil. Drizzle with olive oil and season with salt and pepper. Wrap foil around cauliflower completely, making a purse. There should be no openings.

Roast in oven for 40 to 50 minutes.

Remove from oven and immediately transfer to a medium sized bowl. Add cream cheese. Blend with a handheld immersion blender, or mash with potato masher. Once cream cheese is melted and incorporated throughout, fold in chives.

Serve immediately.

110 calories • 11 g carbohydrate • 5 g fiber • 7 g fat (2 g saturated fat) • 5 g protein • 350 mg sodium

Oven Sweet Potato "Fries"

These "fries" provide more vitamins and calcium and less saturated fat than traditional white potato fries.

Serves 4

Ingredients

4 small sweet potatoes, cut into quarters, then into wedges (about 4 cups)
2 tablespoons extra virgin olive oil
½ teaspoon freshly ground black pepper
¼ teaspoon kosher salt
¼ teaspoon garlic powder

Instructions

Preheat oven to 375°F.

Place potato wedges in large mixing bowl and add remaining ingredients. Toss well, coating each wedge with olive oil and spices.

Spread wedges in an even layer on a large baking pan. Bake 30 minutes or until potatoes start to brown on edges.

110 calories • 12 g carbohydrate • 2 g fiber • 7 g fat (1 g saturated fat) • <1 g protein • 170 mg sodium

Mushroom and Barley Risotto

This version of an Italian classic provides more
fiber and protein without skimping on flavor.

Serves 4

Ingredients

3 cups low sodium
vegetable broth

1 cup water

1 cup quick cooking barley

1 tablespoon plus 1 teaspoon
canola oil

½ cup white onion, finely
chopped

1 tablespoon minced garlic

1 ½ cups baby portabella
mushrooms, roughly
chopped

½ cup dry white wine

¼ teaspoon freshly ground
black pepper

1 tablespoon lemon zest

2 tablespoons finely grated
parmesan cheese

½ cup Italian flat leaf parsley,
finely chopped

Instructions

Combine vegetable broth and
water in a small sauce pan. Heat
until warm.

In a separate large sauté pan,
toast barley over medium-high
heat until golden brown (about
2 minutes), stirring constantly.
Transfer barley to bowl and
set aside.

In the same sauté pan, add
canola oil and onion. Cook
until translucent. Add garlic
and mushrooms. Cook 1 minute.
Add white wine and barley and
cook until most of wine has
evaporated, stirring constantly.

Using a ladle, pour in ½ cup
of warm vegetable broth and
reduce heat to medium. Once
barley has absorbed liquid,
add another ½ cup of vegetable broth, stirring occasionally.
Repeat this step until all broth is
used. Add black pepper, lemon
zest, and parmesan cheese.
Stir well.

Remove from heat and stir in
fresh parsley. Serve immediately.

Tip

▸ Risotto should be thick and not watery.

▸ Different varieties of mushrooms can be substituted for the baby portabellas.

▸ Frequent stirring will prevent risotto from sticking to bottom of pan.

220 calories • 33 g carbohydrate • 5 g fiber • 6 g fat (1 g saturated fat) • 7 g protein • 220 mg sodium

Parmesan Herb Spaghetti Squash

A spaghetti-like side dish with a fraction of the carbohydrates of regular pasta.

Serves 4

Ingredients

- **1** spaghetti squash, cut in half length wise
- **1** cup water
- **1** tablespoon extra virgin olive oil
- **½** teaspoon freshly ground black pepper
- **⅛** teaspoon kosher salt
- **1** tablespoon fresh parsley, roughly chopped
- **2** tablespoons grated parmesan cheese

Instructions

In a microwave-safe dish, place squash cut side up. Pour water in the bottom of the dish and wrap tightly with plastic wrap. Microwave 10 to 12 minutes or until squash is easily comes away from outer skin. Uncover and allow squash to sit 5 minutes.

Using a fork, scrape squash into a medium serving dish. Drizzle with olive oil and mix in remaining ingredients.

Serve immediately.

Tip

► For a nuttier flavor, roast the squash in the oven. Rub cut side of squash with olive oil and place face down on a baking sheet. Bake at 375°F for 45 minutes to 1 hour.

110 calories • 16 g carbohydrate • 3 g fiber • 4.5 g fat (1 g saturated fat) • 3 g protein • 400 mg sodium

Green Beans with Almonds

Say good-bye to boring green beans! This simple side dish provides a great flavor to your meal and is sure to be a trusted favorite.

Serves 6

Ingredients

1 pound of green beans, washed and trimmed
¼ teaspoon kosher salt
1 tablespoon good quality extra virgin olive oil
2 cloves garlic, chopped
⅓ cup slivered almonds

Instructions

Bring a large pot of water to a boil. Add green beans. Cook for 5 minutes. Drain beans in colander and rinse with cold water. Set aside.

Return pot to heat. Add olive oil and garlic. Sauté over low heat for 2 to 3 minutes. Add almonds and sauté 5 more minutes. Add beans and salt. Mix well. Serve immediately.

Tip

▸ Rinsing with cold water cools the beans and stops them from cooking. It also retains the bright green color of the beans.

75 calories • 7 g carbohydrate • 3 g fiber • 5 g fat (< 1 g saturated fat) • 3 g protein • 320 mg sodium

Citrus Avocado Side Salad

This sweet salad is loaded with healthy fats, vitamin C and other antioxidants.

Serves 4

Ingredients

- ½ small red onion, thinly sliced
- **3** cups baby kale leaves
- **2** cups Brussels sprouts, shredded
- **1** avocado, sliced
- **2** cara cara or navel oranges, peeled
- **1** tablespoon extra virgin olive oil
- **2** tablespoons white wine vinegar
- **1** teaspoon honey
- ⅛ teaspoon kosher salt
- ¼ teaspoon freshly ground black pepper
- ¼ cup feta cheese, crumbled

Instructions

Soak onion slices in a small bowl of ice water while you prepare salad.

In a large shallow bowl, add kale and Brussels sprouts. Top with avocado and orange sections.

In a small bowl, whisk together olive oil, vinegar, honey, salt, and pepper. Set aside.

Remove onions from water and add to salad. Sprinkle with crumbled feta. Drizzle with dressing and let sit for 5 to 10 minutes before serving to soften kale and Brussels sprouts.

Tip

► If you can't find baby kale, you can substitute other greens such as spinach or arugula.

190 calories • 22 g carbohydrate • 7 g fiber • 11 g fat (2.5 g saturated fat) • 6 g protein • 230 mg sodium

Sautéed Garlicky Spinach

This quick side dish is packed with fiber and nutrients from iron-rich spinach. The combination with garlic and red pepper gives it a nice kick.

Serves 2

Ingredients

1 ½ teaspoon of good quality
  extra virgin olive oil
1 clove of garlic, chopped
Pinch of dried red pepper flakes
4 cups washed spinach
  (about 5 ounces)
Pinch of salt

Instructions

In a sauté pan, warm olive oil over low heat. Add garlic and red pepper flakes. Sauté on medium heat until golden brown.

Add spinach and salt. Sauté over medium-high heat until spinach has wilted (about 3 to 4 minutes).

Serve immediately.

48 calories • 3 g carbohydrate • 7 g fiber • 4 g fat (0 g saturated fat) • 2 g protein • 134 mg sodium

Roasted Asparagus

This savory roasted asparagus is a good source of folate, vitamins A, C, E, and K, as well as chromium.

Serves 3

Ingredients

1 pound asparagus spears
3 cloves of garlic,
    roughly chopped
1 tablespoon extra virgin olive oil
½ teaspoon freshly ground
    black pepper
¼ teaspoon kosher salt

Instructions

Preheat oven to 350°F.

Trim ends off of asparagus spears, about 1 inch. Spread evenly on a large baking sheet. Toss with olive garlic, olive oil, salt, and pepper.

Roast 15 to 20 minutes or until ends are brown and crispy.

70 calories • 7 g carbohydrate • 3 g fiber • 4.5 g fat (0.5 g saturated fat) • 4 g protein • 200 mg sodium

Corn on the Cobb
with Cilantro Lime Butter

This infused butter is so easy and gives
regular old corn on the cobb a zesty bite.

Serves 4

Ingredients

4 ears corn, shucked

Cilantro Lime Butter:
4 tablespoons unsalted butter,
   at room temperature
1 teaspoon chopped
   cilantro leaves
1 teaspoon lime zest
Juice from half a lime
¼ teaspoon salt

Instructions

Place corn in a large pot of
unsalted boiling water. Cover
the pot and return it to a boil.
Cook the corn for 5 to 7 minutes
or until tender. Remove from heat.

Put the butter in a small mixing
bowl. Using a rubber spatula, mix
in the cilantro, zest, juice, and salt.
Use immediately or refrigerate up
to 5 days.

Serve each ear of corn with 1
tablespoon cilantro lime butter.

Tip

▸ To grill corn, pull silks off, but keep husks on. Soak ears of corn
in a large bowl of cold water with 1 tablespoon of salt for 10
minutes. Place corn on a hot grill and cover. Turn corn every
5 minutes until done.

180 calories • 18 g carbohydrate • 2 g fiber • 13 g fat (7 g saturated fat) • 3 g protein • 54 mg sodium